# KNEES UP MOTHER BROWN

or

# How to Get New Knees and Survive

By Pam Bayfield

–

ISBN 978-0-9579760-2-3



pambayfield@gmail.com



**Disclaimer.**
Whilst every effort has been made to ensure that the information contained in this book was correct at the time of publication, no liability will be accepted by the author for the accuracy or completeness of the information. To the best of the author's knowledge, the material used is free of copyright or has been acknowledged. An apology is extended for the use of any material unwittingly unacknowledged.

Printed and Bound by
Mini-Publishing

www.minipublishing.com.au

**Also by Pam Bayfield**

*To Those Who Wait*
*From Ochre To Azure Blue (autobiography)*
*Anneke's Story - Anna Van der Laarse*
*A Leading Lady – The Story of Mary Jolly*
*Silver Dreams - Story Of Broken Hill*
*Come With Me – The Story Of Joan Fisher*
*Challenging Lives- The Story of Paula and Julien Vanslambrouck*
*For the Love of Grace – A Story of Love and Betrayal*
*For the Love of Grace – The Sequel*
*For the Love of Grace – The Next Generation*
*The Doug Nolan Story – a navigator on a Catalina.*
*A Country Boy At Heart – Arthur McKenzie*
*For the Love of Grace – The Aftermath*
*For the Love of Grace – The Finale*

CONTENTS

## DEDICATION

This book is dedicated to the wonderful doctors and nurses who helped me through my bilateral knee operation and who help so many others in the same boat.

## ACKNOWLEDGEMENTS

There are many people to thank in writing this book. Of course I want to thank my doctor Dr William K Walter and all the other doctors who helped me during my stay at the Mater Hospital. A big thank you to the wonderful nurses who cared for me so well and gave me encouragement when I was feeling so miserable. To all the people at Delmar, the rehab hospital in Dee Why I want to say a big thank you. To Josie, my physio you were a great help and with your gentle persuasion made me go that extra mile to get my knees to bend.

There are some others I would especially like to thank. Tom Gray, my masseur visited me in my misery when my back was playing up and helped ease the pain. Margaret Goulding, my hairdresser visited me twice in hospital and made me feel human again and a little more presentable. Margaret Sheumack came with me on my first visit to Dr Walter and supported me every inch of the way. Thanks to all my tennis buddies who sent flowers and cards and visited me in hospital; it was you who gave me the inspiration to work hard to be able to join you once more on the tennis court.

To all my other friends thank you for your phone calls and messages via the e-mail and letters. It is comforting to know people care. To my family I give my biggest thank you. You put up with my moaning and groaning but gave me encouragement to get better as quickly as I could.

Thank you Dr Cross for allowing me to use your name in one of the stories from my e-mailers and information on your website and a research paper you sent me. Thank you for reading the manuscript. Your name was mentioned many times by grateful patients whom you have helped with your skill and expertise. Thank you for introducing me to Dr Greg Roger at Australian Surgical Design who showed me how the prothesis is made. Thank you to my doctor Dr Bill Walter who kindly offered to read the manuscript and made helpful comments.

Thank you Erika Oller and publisher Jeremy Black for allowing me to use your design on my front cover. Thank you to Joan Evans who edited my story and to Robyn McWilliam who did the final edit.

If my book helps one person make up his or her mind to go ahead and have the procedure done then this will have been all worthwhile. Being forewarned is to be forearmed, isn't that the old saying?

## PREFACE

## Quote Dr William K Walter

'In days gone by there were a lot of people sitting on verandahs watching the world go by. With modern **joint replacement** surgery they can remain mobile and pain free and have a good quality of life.'

## STRUCTURE OF THE KNEE

'The knee is a complicated hinged joint. The end of the femur, the large bone of the upper leg which articulates at the hip and extends to the knee, is smoothly rounded off and rests comfortably into the saucer shaped top of the tibia, the long bone that extends from the lower part of the knee to the ankle joint. The surfaces of the bones are covered with cartilage - grisly material attached to the bone and making joint cavities. There are two menisci in the knee which are easily damaged - they stabilize the joint yet still allowing flexibility of movement. These are crescent shaped pads of fibrous cartilage which help take the weight.

In sports injuries the menisci can be torn and need to be removed. Without them the knee can still function, but wear and tear increases so that arthritis may set in later in life. To lubricate the joint, the surfaces are bathed in synovial fluid. This is a clear fluid which lubricates and nourishes all the tissues inside the joint capsule.

Strength and stability are provided by the fibrous bands called ligaments. Without hindering the hinge movement of the knee these ligaments lie on both sides and in the middle of the joint and hold it firmly in place. The movements of the knee are governed by these ligaments and muscles in the thigh. Those in the front, the quadriceps, pull the knee straight and those behind, the hamstrings, hinge it backwards.

To prevent the tendon at the front from rubbing the joint as it moves a bone has been built into the tendon. This bone is the kneecap or patella and lies in the tendon itself, unattached to the rest of the knee. The knee is prone to wear and tear and overuse, as it is both weight bearing and our prime means of movement. When our knees become too painful to walk, we could be confined to a wheelchair, emphasizing why knee surgery is considered the best option to maintain a normal healthy lifestyle.'

Tom Gray June 2005.

Tom is my masseur and has been giving my husband, mother and me a massage once a fortnight for a number of years. Tom deals with sports people and has sport injury experience. I met Tom about seven years ago after struggling with a back problem that wouldn't respond to normal physio and chiropractic treatment. He used the Bowen treatment on me and in two sessions had me fixed. I then went on a two weekly massage and he kept me mobile when my knees were playing up. He kept telling me I should have something done but I held off as long as I could. I wasn't looking forward to getting new knees but in the end it became a necessity.

## What is a Total Knee Replacement?

This explanation is taken from a handout given to patients before they enter hospital. My hospital was the Mater Hospital at Crows Nest, Sydney. Thank you for your permission to use it in my book.

*A total Knee Replacement is an operation that replaces a knee that has been damaged by arthritis or trauma. Your knee joint is a hinge joint at which your thigh bone (femur) articulates with your shin bone (tibia). The joint is surrounded by cartilage, muscles and ligaments. Arthritis occurs when the cartilage lining the joint is worn away exposing the underlying bone. The joint becomes rough and distorted, resulting in pain and restricted movement.*

*The total Knee Replacement is a prosthesis which has the same basic parts as your own knee. There is a femoral component which replaces the worn end of the femur and a tibial component. There is a plastic spacer between these two components. These new components may be cemented or non-cemented depending on the type of prosthesis recommended by your doctor.*

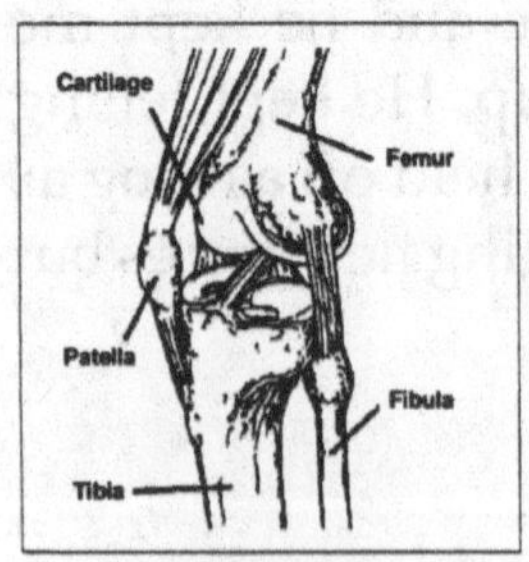

Normal Knee

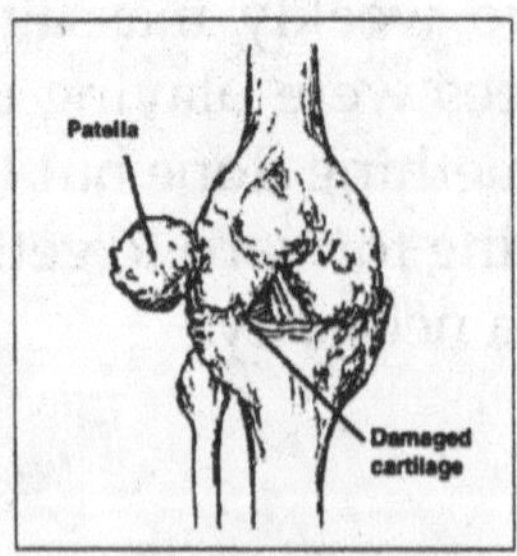

Osteoarthritis of the Knee

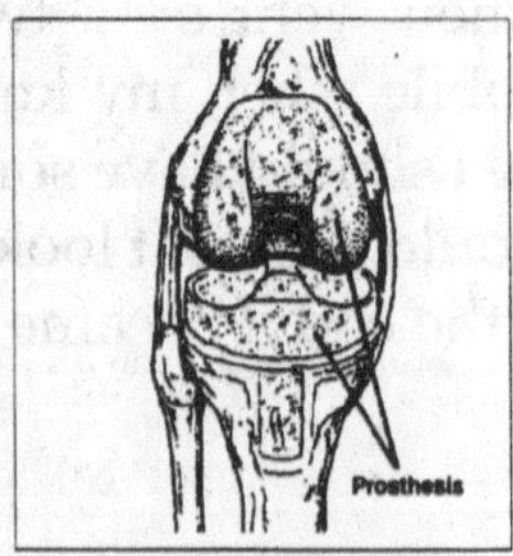

Total Knee Replacement

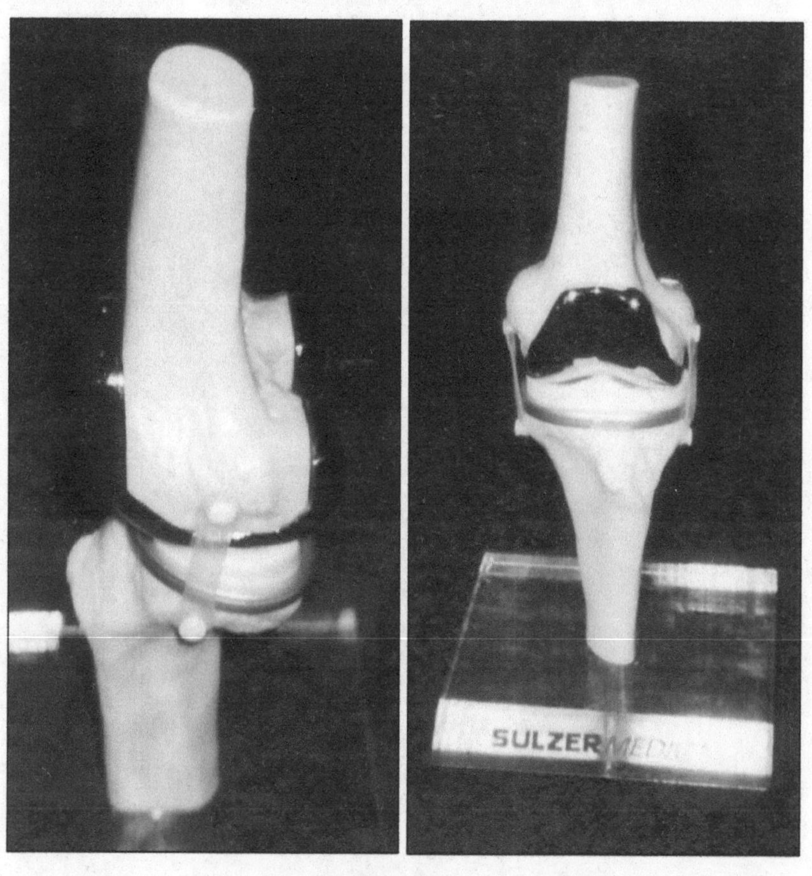


**This is how the prosthesis looks from different angles.**

## PROLOGUE

On 29 July 2004 I had a bilateral knee operation at the Mater Hospital. My doctor was Dr William K Walter. If I had known that there was a chance of things going wrong I may not have gone ahead but then again how could I put up with a knee that went in its own strange direction and another that could hardly get up steps. After reading many e-mails from fellow bilateral patients I realized that some were extremely pleased with their new knees and others not so happy. How did I find this out? I placed a piece in the "*Insearch*" column of the Daily Telegraph in April 2005 nine months after my operation. This is what I wrote:-

### *PEOPLE WITH NEW KNEES*

> *I would like to contact any people with new knees to see how they are progressing. I'm writing a story about my experiences and would like to compare with others who have been through the same operation especially ones who had two done at once like myself. E-mail me on …………. I put in my e-mail address.*

I was astounded with the response. After reading their emails I realized how much better I felt about myself but this one really shocked me.

*Hi Pam*

*I had both knees replaced on 8 September 2003 and I was in hospital for 17 days. The maximum bend I could get was about 40 degrees. On 12 November, 2003 I was admitted again for six days and had both knees manipulated. They both seized up again with a maximum bend of about 40 degrees even though they were bent to 110 degrees while under anaesthetic. Admitted again on 21 November 2003 for 11 days where they did a revision on both knees and again being bent to 110 degrees while under anaesthetic. This time they removed scar tissue from the joints. The knees seized again to a maximum of 50 degrees. On 15/4/2004 I visited the North Shore Sports Clinic and saw a knee specialist and he stated that calcification had set in and advised me to go onto anti-inflammatories. On 18 August 2004 revision again on the right knee and again bent under anaesthetic and bent to 110 degrees. This time they took scar tissue and calcification out of the knee. After 10 days being in hospital, there was still no improvement in the knees. As it is now some 20 months since the first operation, I am still unable to walk unaided. I use a walking stick. Both knees are very stiff but virtually pain free. The right knee seems to want to give away at times. The last time I saw my doctor, apparently the prosthesis that was used was faulty and there is a class action being taken against the manufacturer.*
*Greg Pearce*

My God, if I'd read this before my operation I would have run a thousand miles. However after reading the next one I would have been heartened to go ahead.

*Hi Pam,*

*I noticed your request for information on double knee replacement recipients in last Saturday's Daily Telegraph. So, here I am, double knee replacements at the Mater Hospital seven years ago last January, back on the golf course within three months and have never looked back. Sure they are not your own in that they don't bend so far and there are certain restrictions like running etc., but I was in agony before the operation and my knees were governing my life. I trust yours are working for you.*
*Paul Roberts*

I replied to Paul and told him about my experience and he e-mailed me back. He elaborated on his recovery and had a wonderful tale to tell which I will include later in the book. His experience would have given me hope.

Here is another good one.

*Hi Pam*
*I am 77 and my ops were 2001 and 2003. The rehab was a bit tough especially the stationary bike but after a few weeks it was all go. I have no discomfort now. My recreation is playing bridge and I have been in the Australian open team during the last few years. I have a large business here in Cootamundra employing 140 people and interests in Sydney. My ops have kept me mobile and enable me to get around quite comfortably in administering my business. Your intention to write a book about your experiences seems a good idea and it may help people who are concerned at the thought of the operation to go ahead. Keep in touch and let me know how you are going.*
*Regards*
*Barry Noble*

The best letter was from an 85 year old lady who has had her knees for 20 years and they are still going strong. Her determination in finding the young doctor who performed the operation took Rita on a journey of discovery and her story and those of many others will be included later in the book. These e-mails opened my eyes and made me realize how good it is to share experiences with other people who have been through the same trauma. Many a time I would have dearly loved to know if I was going well in comparison with others. Reading about the problems some people encountered made me feel much better about myself.

Why did I want to have my two knees done and how bad were they? I was down to bone on bone in both knees and being a tennis player that was disastrous. My right knee was going further and further off to the right and I hated myself in shorts or a bathing suit. Others in my tennis group had been brave enough to have one knee replaced and one of my friends had the courage to have two done at once. Why did I consider doing the same?

I had been a keen tennis player since I was a young girl. I worked my way up through the grades until I was playing 'A' Grade for Armidale Tennis Club. I represented in team matches with other nearby towns. I also represented Armidale Teachers' College while I was training and when I came to Sydney I played competition for a number of years at Manly Lawn Tennis Club. Tennis has played a big part in my life.

Naturally I did have some knee and ankle problems during that time and the money I spent on chiropractors and physios added up to a small fortune. But that is what everyone did when injury interrupted their time on the court. The sooner we got back playing the better.

My husband Garnet and I decided to build a tennis court in our backyard in the 80s ostensibly for the use of our eldest son Justin who was shaping up as a good player but when he turned 18 he went to university in America on a tennis scholarship. Garnet invited a few friends to play on a Saturday while I was still playing Tuesday and Thursdays for Manly Lawn.

After returning to teaching in 1988 I had to give my competitive tennis away but began inviting friends to play in the holidays on our court. Everyone would bring a plate and we all partook of a delicious lunch after playing all morning. That went on for a number of years until I retired from teaching 10 years later.

Now I could play during the week and I found a group of ladies who wanted to join me. Those were happy times and I looked forward to my tennis day. However, I was beginning to have trouble with my knees and my doctor put me on anti-inflammatories as he said I had arthritis. My right knee ever so slowly began to turn at a funny angle. However, I was not going to give up playing. It got to the stage where I could hardly run on the court and my walking days were over. I knew I had to do something and soon.

A tennis mate, Margaret Sheumack had already been given a new knee and to our surprise was back on the court after three months. She came and played with us a few times and we all remarked how well she was moving. I used to joke and say I wanted a knee just like hers. She had put a lot of effort into her rehabilitation. Another tennis friend, Jan Ryding was going in to have TWO done at once. I followed her progress with much interest. I knew from what she told me it was no fun and she had been through a lot of pain. Before her operation she could hardly walk and her knees had been giving her hell. One tennis day about eight weeks into her rehabilitation she visited us and she was beaming. She was now pain free. Jan had had to bully her doctor into doing both knees. Most doctors like to do one at a time.

Another in our group, Bev Trim decided she had had enough of her bad knee and went to the doctor to see if she could be given a new one. He agreed to do it in Manly Hospital and the day I went to visit she was looking pale and sick. 'This other leg is going to the grave with me, Pam,' Bev told me and I knew what a horrible experience it must be. This was what I was facing. Could I go through with it? All my friends thought I should and not leave it too long. Margaret inspired me to go and see her doctor, Dr Walter and even came to the first appointment with me. He took one look at my deformed leg and agreed to do it. At that point I was only going to have one done. As I had a trip to Norfolk Island booked for a Writers Festival the date was put off until 29 July, about five months away. When I look back that was a silly thing to do as I had too much time to think about it.

About a month before going into hospital I was sitting on my front porch and I began thinking about my left knee. I'll have one good leg and the other will still need doing at some later stage. What good is that? Perhaps I should have them done together. I spoke to Garnet and he said do whatever I wanted. I rang Dr Walter who told me he'd see me with new x-rays. Once he saw them I knew my die was cast.

'Yes, your left knee is not very good. All right, I'll do them both together.'

I told him I was terrified of the operation and his reply was, 'Oh, you'll be all right in a day or two.' Oh doctor, if only!

Chapter 1

# Oh Doctor, if only!

## Day 1 Thursday 29 July 2004

I open my eyes. It's all over. Where's the pain? I can't feel any. I lift my head and see two straight legs in front of me. Hallelujah! How long have I been unconscious? I don't remember a thing after being wheeled into the operating theatre. Only a big black hole. It must be about 2pm and I am back in my room. I had gone in at 7am to be the first cab off the rank. A nurse is hovering over me, asking how I am feeling. I feel fine. I had been given a spinal block to dull the pain. This isn't going to be too bad after all.

I am attached to drips and have a catheter in. My knees are draining and I'm told I have lost a lot of blood and was given three transfusions. At that point I didn't care. I could have had my throat cut and it wouldn't have mattered. I am in another world, drifting in and out of sleep. Natalie, my nurse is never far from my side. To have such a caring girl on my first day is wonderful. I do remember Dr Walter looking in and when I see him I call out, 'Doctor, you're my hero.' He has a funny look on his face and must have thought I was delirious.

I bet he said to his staff out of earshot, 'She won't think that tomorrow,' and by golly I didn't.

## Day 2 Friday 30 July

Today the pain starts. The epidural has worn off and my knees are now letting me know that something major has been done to them. The anesthetist has to be called in to give me a more powerful painkiller in the drip. A little green button is placed in my hand and I'm told to use it whenever I feel the pain. The sister tells me I can't overdose no matter how many times I push it. That green button was given a good workout that day. Oh God, I am feeling so nauseous! I can't stand the look of food. It's going to be a long day but as I lie on my back I doze on and off. I am awoken every hour during the night for my blood pressure to be taken and to see to the drips. How is a poor girl supposed to sleep? As well they attach a pump to both legs which pulsates, making it hard to sleep. I'm told it is to stop clots forming. I am to be given Heparin straight into my stomach for the first few days and then go on Warfarin. This is to be done as a precaution as I'm prone to clotting. I have a wonderful lady doctor, Dr Rosemary Prichard-Davies, looking after me while I'm in hospital. She's an angel. She will be coming every day to monitor my progress.

## Day 3 Saturday 31 July

This is my worst day. I'm feeling ghastly. I know that sooner or later the physiotherapist is going to come and try to get me up. I don't have a clue how I am going to get these two lumps of lead to move. The thought of putting weight on my knees terrifies me. The nurse comes to take out my drips and free me from the bed. This is a big step forward, but it also means I will be getting up soon. Oh hell!

'It's time, Mrs Bayfield. We have to get you up today.' No, go away. Not today. Please not today. 'Now come on, we'll do some simple exercises first. Press your legs into the bed. Good and now can you lift your right leg?'

To my surprise I find that I can lift it a little and this was my crooked leg. What a different story with the other one! It objects right away and doesn't want to move an inch. What is the matter with it? Don't tell me it's now my worst leg! Obviously, it's paying me back for having it done at the last minute.

The physio speaks again, 'I'll help you sit up and then you can swing your legs around to the floor.' The moment of truth! So here I am sitting with my legs dangling over the bed. 'Here is the frame to hold onto, Mrs Bayfield. Put all your weight on your arms and you will be able to support your body.' My head is swimming and the thought of putting my feet to the floor is more than I can manage. I am a chicken.

'You must remember that you have two brand new knees and they are very strong. They will not crumble under you but will support your weight. Now come on, up you get.' With gentle urging I am guided to the frame and onto my feet. They don't feel too bad. I'm supposed to take a few steps but I feel too woozy. I have to sit down or I'll fall in a big heap. 'Never mind, we will try again tomorrow. Lie back and rest.' Thank goodness, she's not going to insist on walking just yet.

That evening I feel desperate. Why, oh why, did I allow this to happen? I can't see how I am going to make it to day four let alone four or five weeks down the track. I ask for a sleeping tablet which thankfully bombs me out until I'm woken for obs.

## Day 4 Sunday 1 August

By my fourth day I am down to taking painkillers with water and no drips. The catheter is still in which means I don't have to get up to go to the toilet. My blood pressure is down and my blood count is low so no wonder I'm feeling drowsy. I'm given my first shower on a stool and a male orderly assists - no modesty allowed. It is wonderful having the warm water flush over my body instead of sponge baths. I'm feeling relieved as the previous night I had been given an enema. The utter joy at being able to move my bowels was immeasurable.

In the afternoon my sons, Cameron and Mark along with my daughter-in law, Nadia come to visit, followed later by Garnet and Mum. Why did they all come on the same day? How am I going to be able to talk to them? I try to sit up for half an hour but it takes so much out of me I have to lie down again. I know they want to see me as soon as possible but I don't feel like talking. I also have a few phone calls from concerned friends and I tell them to come and see me when I go to Delmar, the rehab hospital. I'm feeling so dreadful, how could I possibly be polite to visitors?

## Day 5 Monday 2 August

I am given a smaller frame today and go for a walk using it. I see others charging up and down the hall and wonder what they have had done - surely not two knees! I ask one man and he tells me he had a hip replacement. He is moving so well. Perhaps he'd been in a while and I heard hips aren't as bad as knees anyway. I go to the corner and back and that exhausts me.

Today the nurse takes out my catheter. I have become quite attached to it. It has saved me getting up and down all day. Now it means I have to go to the toilet by myself. I suppose it will be good exercise for these blasted knees! When the icepacks are placed on them they make me want to go more. My knees are given a good work out in the days ahead going backwards and forwards to the bathroom. Thank goodness I have an ensuite so I don't have to go far. The nurses tell me to drink, drink and drink some more. Surely that would make me have to get up more often.

Margaret drops in and I'm very pleased to see her. Having been through the same experience, albeit one knee, she understands my plight. Our mutual friend Norma Moss had gone in the day before at the same hospital and she had a half knee replacement. Margaret is going to visit her as well. Norma is also going to Delmar and I will be following as soon as I'm given the green light. Only having a half knee replacement means her recovery is much quicker than mine.

Margaret understands how difficult it is for me, lying on my back the whole time and having to sleep that way as well. No wonder I had trouble with my back later on. After chatting for a while she leaves to visit Norma and the physio comes to take me for a walk. I don't quite make it around the block. Putting one leg in front of the other is exhausting. I can't wait to get back to bed. From then on it is all downhill. My stomach is bloated and because I feel nauseous, I can't eat any food. The nurse gives me some peppermint water to ease the wind pains which doesn't do much good. I then ask for some tonic water to see if I can burp. A little while later a terrible smell from down the hallway reaches me and that really turns my stomach. Luckily there is a bowl handy. This is the first time I have vomited although I have been feeling so ill.

I settle down after that and watch television. I take a sleeping tablet but have a disturbed sleep. I think I get up about five times to go to the toilet. How I miss the catheter!

## Day 6 Tuesday 3 August

A bad day. I don't feel like lunch as I'm so bound up and want to go to the toilet but can't. The nurse gives me two suppositories but they have no effect. I lie down and try to sleep. My solitude is broken by the physio wanting to take me for a walk on arm crutches.

'Do I have to? Please can't I stay in bed a little longer?'

'No, we're going to try two new walking sticks today. Up you get.' I could murder her. It is the last thing I want to do. I still feel rotten as I haven't been to the toilet. Can't a girl have any peace?

'Left stick forward, right foot forward, right stick forward left foot forward.' She sounds like an army major. I make my slow torturous way down the hall with sympathetic eyes following my every move. Poor woman, the other patients must have thought. My eyes are glued to the carpet and my physio keeps telling me to keep my head up. What and fall over? No way.

I keep going and finally we reach the lounge room at the end of the hall. Inside is a small two way staircase, obviously for practising going up and down.

'You don't expect me to go up those today?' I plaintively cry.

'No, no I just want you to put your foot there on that step and push your knee forward as far as it will go and hold for 15 seconds.'

I try the best I can. Oh, the pain! My right knee doesn't like it too much but my left one hates it even more. I know it's important to get the knees to bend but does it have to be now? As I was informed later the sooner the knee bends the better or the scar tissue will not allow it to bend at all. I then have to walk all the way back again. I feel like keeling over any minute but I battle on until I reach my room. I can't wait to get back into bed. What a wimp!

Surely now I can go to the toilet. But no, I am well and truly clogged. My guardian angel Natalie, the one who nursed me on my first day, comes to my rescue. She gives me two enemas, suitably spaced but nothing works. She gives me a fig concoction which I eat. Yuck! It's horrible. Surely that will do the trick. But no! I wait and wait. Nothing happens. I am up and down to the toilet, giving my new knees a good work out.

I am getting more and more desperate. Finally I take a sleeping tablet and decide to go to sleep. At 4am I am awakened by an urgent need. What a relief to be able to go at last!

I go into a peaceful sleep and when I wake I feel so much better. I can even eat some breakfast. Surely my worst day is over.

## Day 7 Wednesday 4 August

I have to change rooms today as they are going to re-new the carpet. What a time to do it! That is the last thing I want to do but the nurses are wonderful. I don't have to do anything. They just push me to another room and bring all my belongings. I am then sent down for an ultra-sound to see if I have any clots but thankfully there aren't any. The Warfarin is working well.

Catherine Smith, a writing friend comes to visit in the afternoon. She brings me some pretty pink sweet peas and a book to read. She only stays half an hour and by then I'm really tired and fall asleep. When I wake up, I take myself for a walk around the room and almost immediately the physio arrives to take me for a longer walk. Left right, left right, why can't I get it right? By the end I'm beginning to get the hang of it. Will I ever feel normal again? Oh please, let me feel like eating dinner tonight!

I force down two sandwiches and a bowl of ice-cream. I watch a few shows on television before falling asleep. My stomach is much relieved but even so I'm still up and down during the night.

## Day 8 Thursday 5 August

A male nurse helps me have a shower. Well at least he makes sure I'm secure on the chair before letting me use the handheld nozzle to wash myself. The feeling is uplifting. The power of the water, it does wonders. I take myself for a walk and meet another lady who has had a knee done. We commiserate with each other. That sick feeling is still with me. I struggle with lunch.

My friends Barbara and Bruce Obermann come to see me and bring me flowers and chocolates. It's lovely to see them but it is an effort to keep chatting. Barbara can see I'm struggling and they leave after half an hour.

After tea I call the nurse and tell her I'm feeling dreadful. She tells me my blood count is down and that I may need a blood transfusion. No wonder I'm so tired! I may not be going to Delmar tomorrow. At that point of time I couldn't care less.

## Day 9 Friday 6 August

Here I am at day nine and am still weak as a kitten. Oh, to feel my old self again! I wonder what is in store for me today. Dr Prichard-Davies advises the nurses that I won't be going to Delmar until Monday at the earliest. She has been to see me every day and I always look forward to her visits. She tells me I'm not going to get another transfusion but I'm to be given iron tablets to boost my blood count. Surely, I will feel better soon.

'The rest over the weekend will do you good,' she tells me and I don't argue. I know that once I'm at Delmar I'll be expected to begin all those horrible exercises and I don't feel up to it right now. I look in the mirror and see what a mess my hair is. What am I going to do about it? It badly needs washing. Will Margaret Goulding, my hairdresser, come to the hospital and blow dry it for me? I ring her and she agrees. What a sweetheart! I wash it under the shower and wait for her. She makes me feel like a new person. At least now I will look all right if anyone comes to visit. Thank you Margaret!

Hallelujah! I eat all my sandwiches today. They are chicken and mayonnaise and they taste wonderful. It is so good to enjoy eating again. (I realize how much food played a big part in my rehabilitation when I re-read my story). After lunch I go for a walk - still on two crutches - and by the time I come back to my room I'm exhausted. I lie down and listen to some music. Garnet arrives with some clean nighties. I don't know how my dear husband manages to do everything at home and at work and still gets over to see me. His visits are short, in and out. He seems to be coping. Cameron and Nadia invited him for tea one night and he went out with Mark another night. I don't think he's starving. Men are resilient when they have to be.

This hospital is so quiet and peaceful. Thank goodness I came here. It is wonderful seeing the pink ladies come in and water my flowers. No wonder they have lasted so long, with such loving care. The nurses have all been cheerful and helpful. Some are full time nurses while others are only part time. Some are agency nurses who put their names down and ask for specific days and jobs are found for them. All of them are knowledgeable and kind. The night nurses are a special breed and I had some terrific ones.

I'm beginning to think I can get over this and come out the other side. For a while it all seemed too much. I'm even looking forward to dinner.

Here I am at 3am with icepacks on my knees having just had two painkillers, writing in my diary. My bladder keeps getting me up. Good exercise, I suppose. Whenever I can't sleep I put on the radio and listen to soothing music. Usually, I drop back to sleep.

Earlier today I met a young Irish nurse who came out with six friends and they all share a one bedroom flat in the city. They have moved around a lot in the time they've been in Australia, picking up nursing jobs along the way. She tells me they are now splitting up, some going back home and others going further afield. My nurse is contemplating staying as she has met a nice young Aussie sailor. She will certainly be an asset to our country if she decides to stay.

Later in the day I have a long talk with a male nurse and I ask him why he decided to do nursing. He tells me he didn't get enough marks to get into his first choice of physiotherapy. One of his brother's friends is a nurse and convinced him to give it a go. There were only 15 blokes out of his class of 60. He tells me how he was worried about the ribbing he thought he might get and that it was daunting at first. As the course progressed, he began to make friends and began to feel at ease. Now he doesn't give it a thought as he has been nursing for a few years. He says the course is not overly difficult and that a lot of it is common sense. He enjoyed the six to seven weeks of practical nursing in hospitals where he was partnered with a facilitator who showed him how to do things. The hardest thing he found was time management trying to get through all the tasks each day. He tells me the main problem with nursing is the burn out factor with shift work getting a lot of nurses down. I really enjoyed my talk with him.

## Day 10 Saturday 7 August

After eating a good breakfast and showering I'm tired already and the day hasn't started. Oh, to have more energy! When I feel up to it I take myself for a walk around the ward. I get back and my knees are hurting so I ask for some ice and painkillers. There is tennis on television and that keeps my mind off my knees. They are really paining today so I call a nurse who gives me a different painkiller. I try to nod off but am disturbed by a phone call. It is my son Cameron ringing to see how I am. I speak to Nadia as well and then try to get back to sleep but no luck.

I become very emotional today. A compassionate nurse catches me at a vulnerable time. I can't get comfortable and my back is hurting. She sets up my pillows and I start to cry. It suddenly all becomes too much. Out pour my woes and she listens.

'It will get better,' she promises as she pats me on the arm. I cheer up after she goes out. Get over it. There are people worse off than you. I pick up my crutches and proceed down the corridor. I notice a woman lying with two ice packs on her knees. Another bilateral. I stop to talk to her. She is so cheerful telling me she is going home tomorrow but that is not what I want to hear. I suppose I wanted someone to commiserate with so I walk away and return to my room. Tears have begun welling in my eyes on the way back and by the time I reach my room I'm crying again. At that precise moment Mum rings and I sob to her.

She is not very sympathetic and says, 'Don't be so stupid, you've only been there a week.' That is too much. I hang up and cry some more.

My kind nurse appears and says, 'You should have had a visitor today. You've been by yourself too long.'

Stupid me had told my friends not to come and I now realize I do need company. I need someone to jolly me out of my misery. I must ring Garnet and tell him to come tomorrow. A writing friend, Mary Cottam rings after tea and we have a long chat. I need to get a lot of things off my chest and she listens. I have come to the realisation that it is your visitors that cheer you up and help you through the worst of it. I have another disturbed night. At least when I'm asleep, I don't notice my aching back.

## Day 11 Sunday 8 August

Here I am at 6am, sitting up trying to relieve my throbbing back and writing my journal. I've done my exercises and I'm going to make sure I see the physio today. I haven't seen her for a few days. I want her to tell me how I'm progressing and she might have a solution for my sore back. Another day at the Mater to get through before I go to Delmar. This has been a long painful journey but each day is one I won't have to endure again. It must get better.

After my shower I watch some tennis on TV. I'm too tired to go for a walk. Garnet pops in and brings me some e-mails he's printed off. Reading the kind messages cheers me up. He stays for an hour and we have time to chat and I tell him how I'm feeling. Before he goes I decide to show him how I can walk and he follows me around the corridors. Lunch appears as he leaves. Chicken and mayonnaise sandwiches! I enjoy them and realise I have cutlets to look forward to the next day. On Day 3 I had them and they were so delicious I ate every bit even though I wasn't feeling the least like eating at that point.

Listening to music on Radio 2CH is pleasant and I lie back and doze off. My sleep is disturbed by Tim, a different physio to the one I'd been seeing. We go through the exercises and then he takes me for a walk and shows me how to use the crutches so I can go a bit faster. We sail into the lounge room and oh no, the steps! Tim wants me to climb the steps today. He shows me how and I amaze myself by doing it quite well.

I am proud of my efforts. Back in the room he asks me to sit in a chair and pull each knee back as far as it will go. That hurt! He then leaves me with two knees propped on two pillows on another chair. This is meant to straighten my legs. That also hurt! I'm instructed to stay there for ten minutes and then call the nurse. At seven minutes I have had enough and I disentangle myself and get back into bed. Enough is enough!

Mark rings later. It's nice to know my sons are concerned about me. He tells me that Justin who lives in America had rung to ask how I was going. That made me feel good. Pam Gibb, a teaching friend who lives in Yamba rings a bit later. I hadn't told her I was having two knees done and she was quite surprised. Another friend from Mackay, Jeanette Campbell rings after tea and we chat. She sympathises as she had a serious back operation about two years ago. She tells me she can't remember the pain now. I hope that happens to me.

Chapter 2

# Bend Those Knees

## Day 12 Monday 9 August

I should be going to Delmar today. I've had a restless night and my back is painful. I'm told to be ready by 10am. Garnet comes to pick me up but then we're told the bed at Delmar isn't ready and that we can go after lunch. Poor Garnet has to go all the way home and then come back for me. At least I can have cutlets for lunch so I wasn't too disappointed. When they appear they didn't taste as good as the previous ones. Funny about that!

We leave about 1.30pm and Garnet delivers me to the front desk in a wheelchair. A writing friend Jenny Cole-Clark is walking in the door to visit me, not knowing that today is my first day here. The timing couldn't be worse. I'm feeling sick and I don't want Jenny to hang around while I fill out all the paperwork. She decides to leave and I'm grateful. Garnet follows the nurse and me around to my room. Not as big as the Mater. Garnet helps me unpack and then leaves.

The nurse returns to ask more questions and gives me a heat pack for my back. That feels wonderful and gives me instant relief. I must admit I'm not looking forward to another week of agony! Will this time ever end?

## Day 13 Tuesday 10 August

At last daylight comes after an uncomfortable night. I have only slept in snatches and I stayed up late watching television. Anything to take my mind off my discomfort. I'm offered a shower before breakfast and I dress in shorts and a top. That feels better. My back is still aching and in desperation I ring my masseur Tom Gray to see if he can come and help me. He says he'll come at 5pm but can I last till then?

The hospital masseur comes in the morning and gives me a massage of my shoulder and neck so I stupidly cancel Tom. Big mistake! By 4.30pm I'm in trouble. I ring Tom to see if he's home. No answer. He rings back later in the evening and arranges to come the next day. I suppose that's better than nothing. I am feeling so miserable.

Earlier that day I had been for some exercises at the gym and that nearly killed me. Trying to get my knees to bend was excruciating! How am I going to last the distance? This is murder!

Two friends, Jocelyn Alexander and Robyn McWilliam come to visit me, one after the other and although it is wonderful to see them I am finding it hard to keep the conversation going. I finally have to ask each one to leave. By this time my back is throbbing. What else can I expect having to lie like this for so long? Margaret pops in with an inflatable cushion. What an angel! I'm sure that will help.

## Day 14 Wednesday 11 August

It is now a fortnight since the operation. The time has dragged. Each day takes forever. I'm propped up in bed waiting for breakfast. I'm going to my first water therapy in the heated pool soon. My stitches didn't have to come out as they are dissoluble ones and the nurse puts a waterproof spray on the two scars. I'm sure the warm water will be wonderful.

An hour later I am feeling like a new person. I've finished in the pool. It was full of men and women with all sorts of problems, doing gentle exercises in the heated water. When I finally stepped in it felt like heaven - so warm and not too deep. When my two scars were noticed I was told I was brave having two done at once. I don't know about being brave, maybe stupid. Being tall I found I could stand easily in the deep end. I loved every minute of the session. We knew from the gym what exercises to do and amazingly they didn't hurt nearly as much in the water.

When I arrive back in my room Tom has arrived to give me a massage. Oh the joy of it! I lie on my stomach and Tom works on me. It feels so good. Thank you Tom! Lunch follows and it is roast lamb, roast potatoes and pumpkin. I'm starving and eat every bit. It is so good to be hungry again! After lunch I decide to have a sleep as I'd had a big morning but at 1.30pm the physio comes to see if I would like to come around to the gym. You have to be kidding! But I can't very well say no.

Men and women are doing all sorts of exercises on various pieces of equipment. I go through the routine and feel fine. The physios are very helpful and encouraging and don't push you too hard but make it perfectly clear how important it is to get your knees to bend. That is the killer. Ninety degrees is our first aim and then hopefully try to improve on that. One lady I met in the pool just couldn't get her knee to bend and had to go under anesthetic for the doctor to do it for her. She was still having trouble when I met her later.

Faye Rogan, another tennis friend is waiting to see me when I arrive back in my room. We chat for a while and then Jocelyn arrives. My back is really beginning to ache and I suggest we go out into the front foyer. I don't last long before wanting to lie down again. This is such a nuisance. I say goodbye to my visitors and can't wait to lie on my stomach for a little relief. Jan arrives, another bilateral. She knows exactly what I'm going through. In her hand is a punnet of strawberries. I'll be able to have those with my ice-cream each day, I thought. It is great talking to her and we compare notes. She had given me good advice before the operation and because of her, I opted to get two done at once. If she could do it, so could I.

Just as she leaves, Mark walks in. Talk about a busy afternoon. I love seeing my sons and it's comforting that they are so concerned about me. Tea arrives not long after he leaves. Another night to get through but I'm going to take sleeping tablets to help get me off to sleep. I find taking half gives me about three hours sleep before I have to get up to the toilet and then I take the other half. The night goes by much quicker.

## Day 15 Thursday 12 August

What will this day bring? After breakfast I shuffle on crutches down to the pool. I greet the other patients. Everyone is so friendly. We enjoy being able to move in the water which is around 35 degrees. It's like being in a beautiful bath. I'm tired after an hour of walking up and down, bending my knees, bobbing up and down and talking but it's worth it to feel good afterwards. Being able to talk with others who have had knee or hip operations is therapeutic. I realise there are others worse off than I am. However, there are not too many bilaterals.

I finally find one. His name is Michael and we talk every time he comes for his pool session. He tells me what to expect in the weeks ahead. He is about 12 weeks into rehab. He confirms that he also has one knee better than the other and tells me that often happens. It is funny that my crooked leg is now the better one and the knee I decided to have done at the last minute is the worst one. Right from the start my left knee didn't want to lift or bend or do anything it was asked to do without a struggle. It feels much heavier than my right. I can always feel something there and it won't bend as far as the right.

Garnet pops in to take a photo of me in the pool and is going to come back later to take more of me doing exercises. I thought if ever I write a book about my operation, I want some photos as evidence. Once back in my room I shower and rest. I'm exhausted. The phone rings and it is a tennis friend, Nola Munro. She had sent me a funny card with a tennis player bending one knee over the net. The minute I saw it I said, 'Knees up Mother Brown' and knew it would make a wonderful cover for the book I might write one day. I tell her about my progress and then Carolyn Robens comes to visit with a begonia in a pot. It is very pretty. She stays for half an hour and Annette Polman, another friend from Bunka drops in with a sheep skin rug for my poor aching back. It is beautiful to lie on and I really appreciate her bringing it. She stays and chats while I eat my lunch of roast chicken and mashed potatoes.

Just as Annette leaves, I ask for some of my strawberries to go with the ice-cream and chocolate sauce. The nurse had put them in the patient's fridge to keep them cool the day before. They are delicious. At 1.30pm I walk around to the gym and begin the exercises. Garnet arrives and snaps me doing some of them. What a pained expression I must have on my face! It's hard to smile when you're in agony.

After the exercises I fall into bed thoroughly exhausted and go to asleep. When I awake it is nearly five o'clock. Where has the afternoon gone? I now have indigestion and call for the nurse. She sits and talks to me. Finding a nurse with time to talk to her patients is an absolute joy! She explains to me about my bladder problems at night and encourages me to drink more during the day. She also explains how I should be breathing out through my stomach and releasing all the tension. I do this a few times and find I'm getting emotional again as she continues talking to me. She also advises me to sit in the sun each day for about ten minutes to stop depression setting in. I appreciate all her advice. She's a honey!

When she leaves I go for a walk and I practise my breathing when I return. It certainly helps.

## Day 16 Friday 13 August

I had a restless night with not much sleep. Lying in the one position all the time is not helping my back problem. I decide to wash my hair and Margaret, my hairdresser is coming to blow dry it for me. That will lift my spirits. I arrive at the pool with my fashionable hairdo but I don't care. It looks so much better than if I'd done it myself. (Thank you Margaret, you don't know how much I appreciated your visits.)

I feel quite euphoric in the pool. The water feels so good and it does wonders for my morale. I meet Michael again and he tells me he's pleased with his progress. I have to keep looking ahead, he tells me. He says he comes to the pool to help the knee that is not as good as the other one. He is now walking quite long distances and feeling good at the end of it. Oh Michael, you are my inspiration but as yet I can't imagine myself at three months. It seems such a long way off.

Having to wear those wretched tight white stockings is a nuisance but essential to keep blood clots away. I can't put them on myself so a nurse comes to do it for me. She then gives me two bags of ice for my knees and a heat pack for my back. What more could a girl want! I look at myself in the mirror and see my beautiful hair and it gives me such a lift. Oh, the little things in life that make you feel good!

It is cottage pie for lunch and I enjoy it and for sweets I eat six of Jan's strawberries with ice-cream. Such indulgence! I have to move after lunch to the rehab ward W1. I don't have to do a thing. The nurses do all the moving. They certainly earn their money. Now my friends won't know where to find me, so the nurse leaves a notice on the door of my old room. My brother David said he'd call in and Tom is coming to give me a massage. My back is still giving me trouble.

David rushes in 15 minutes before Tom is due. Typical! We can only have a quick chat before he has to go. The massage is heaven and I feel so much better after it. Thanks Tom, you are a life saver! Just as he leaves Joan Evans, another writing friend arrives and we talk for a while. I walk her to the front door showing off my walking skills. Having visitors does lift my spirits and I thank all my friends for their kindness while I was in hospital. The day goes so slowly if no one comes but on most days I had at least one visitor.

The Olympics are coming up so if I'm awake during the night I'll have something to watch. Oh good, afternoon tea is arriving. Another distraction! Tea is soup and sandwiches and I enjoy those. Cameron and Mark arrive not long after tea. It is lovely to see these two handsome men stride into my room. They are going to have pizza together after visiting me. We chat for a while and then they leave.

My sleeping tablet keeps me asleep until 2.30am. Oh good, the Opening Ceremony is about to begin. I watch until all the teams begin appearing and then go back to sleep.

## Day 17 Saturday 14 August

I fill out my menu for Sunday and yippee I'm having roast pork and apple sauce. It looks as if they're in no hurry to kick me out so by staying, I'll hopefully get stronger day by day. I can't believe I have been in hospital 17 days. My scars are looking good and everyone tells me how well I am going and how brave I was to have both knees done at once. I don't know about that. Would I do it again? Maybe not, knowing what I know now. The only thing I'm happy about is that I don't have to go back to have the other one done. I suppose it's better to get the agony all over at once than drag it out over two or three years. Some of the people I met in the pool will have to return to have their other knee done. Poor buggers! I'm better to be here in rehab where they are looking after me, than be a pain in the bum at home. I must get stronger before tackling the back steps.

After breakfast I head for the pool as I know Catherine is coming to see me afterwards. The time in the pool is so beneficial as my knees are really stiff today. The warm water instantly makes them feel better. Everyone smiles as they step into the pool. I can only imagine how cold my pool at home is at this time. It will be quite a while before it will be warm enough for me to go in. I spend 45 minutes doing gentle exercises while talking to other patients. One lady is trying to lose weight, another has had a shoulder operation, others with new knees and hips; all trying to improve their mobility. The heated pool is a god send. The physios give each person his or her personal exercises to do.

I put my dressing gown on and head back to shower in my own room. Catherine will be here any minute. Sure enough she pops her head around the door just as I'm finishing dressing. It's good to see her. We get along well and she always cheers me up. I head back to the gym after she leaves. The exercise I hate the most is the leg lift with the other one bent, lying on my back. My left leg hates bending. The knee bends on the staircase are no fun either. This is where I try to make my knee bend as far as it will go and the physio takes a measurement of the angle. Some days it's better than others. It always bends further after being in the pool.

I'm not ready to tackle the bike yet. Others in my group can use it but I'll get on it when I'm ready. Josie explains that after I'm discharged from Delmar I'll be coming back for about six weeks to do gym and pool, courtesy of my health fund. I can then buy more time in the pool if I want. Yes please, I like the pool!

The gym and pool are closed on Sundays so tomorrow will be a long day. Oh well, time to give my poor aching back a rest. It is still sore and I suppose the exercises are not helping. Lunch of chicken fillet supreme is delicious and I finish off my strawberries with ice-cream and chocolate flavouring. Delectable! I deserve it for what I'm going through at the moment.

The afternoon slips away. I watch a re-play of the Olympic opening ceremony; then a sit in the sun. Bev comes to see me and it is good to chat to someone who understands my predicament. Jocelyn comes again as Bev leaves. No sooner has she left than tea arrives. I even allow myself the indulgence of a glass of wine. At least I have the Olympics to watch to take my mind off my knees and back. I watch until 8pm and then take a sleeping tablet. Perhaps if I'm lucky I'll wake around the time of the swimming finals.

This is what happens. I see Ian Thorpe pip Grant Hackett at the post. A remarkable swim! The 100m Aussie girls win the gold medal for the relay. Wow! I'm glad I was awake to see that. I fall asleep and waken around 6am in time to see the diving. It is quite a cool day.

## Day 18 Sunday 15 August

Today is my mother's birthday. She is 92 years old. I have asked Garnet to buy a small sponge cake and bring it up with her in the afternoon. My brother didn't want to take her out as he wants to watch the Olympics. He is such a sports freak. It will be a long day as the gym and pool are closed. I must do the exercises by myself. Do I have to?

The morning goes quickly and lunch of roast pork arrives. My mouth waters. Looking out the window it is blowing a gale and the temperature in my room drops. I add another layer to the covers on my bed. After lunch I go for a walk to find a warmer room as mine faces away from the sun. Mum and Garnet will be here soon. I hope I feel up to their visit.

I needn't have worried as the time goes quickly and we have a piece of cake with a cup of tea. Mum is happy and thinks I look well. I show her how I can walk and she is impressed. I sit in my chair and I last the distance without having to lie down. A big step forward! I watch some more Olympics before tea. Thank goodness for television and how fortunate that I have something interesting to watch. It fills in the time before going to sleep.

## Day 19 Monday 16 August

I'm still in hospital. My legs are feeling uncomfortable and I try to move them around in bed. Everything is an effort. It rained in the night. We need it badly. I must go and have my shower before venturing down to the pool. My legs feel stiff and need loosening up.

The pool is wonderful and the room has steamed up as it is cold outside. I see my friend Norma and we compare notes. The rehab doctor comes to see me after I return from the pool and says I can go home on Wednesday. Only two more days in hospital! My spirits lift and I tend to overdo the exercises at the gym after lunch. Now I'm suffering with my back. Blast!

I can't imagine what it will be like going home. Will I be able to manage? Where will I find it comfortable to sit? I've already organised a high toilet seat and crutches. Garnet will pick them up tomorrow. The physio has told me the days I'm to come back. I also bought $120 worth of pool vouchers which means I can come back for 10 extra sessions after my regular ones are used up. My fund should pay the cost I'm told.

I call for some ice and a heat pack. My back is really complaining. The heat is soothing and makes me feel better. I suppose this will be the pattern when I get home. Heat and ice. Ice and heat. Tea arrives and I enjoy a pork salad. More television and more Olympics. I take half my sleeping pill and I waken at 2.30am in time to watch Ian Thorpe win GOLD against his archrivals. So exciting! I go back to sleep after the swimming and the tea lady wakens me with a cup of tea. Another day at Delmar.

## Day 20 Tuesday 17 August

When I arrive at the pool I'm the only one there. I have it to myself for 15 minutes. Heaven! I do all my exercises and then more people arrive. It's amazing what benefit this heated pool gives to so many people. The look of pleasure as they enter the water and then the walking up and down begins. Some stay at the wall doing the exercises ever so gently. Some stop to chat and we exchange pleasantries. Everyone is friendly and they all have a story to tell. It is therapeutic to listen to other people's troubles and realise you're not on your own.

I leave the pool and shower and Catherine arrives and we chat. The time goes by quickly. No time to think of my sore back and sore knees. Lunch is chicken schnitzel and it is delicious. I'm enjoying the food at Delmar and it is so good to feel like eating again.

I've been able to tell friends that ring me that I'm going home soon. They have all done so much keeping up my morale. I really want to thank them all. It's nearly three weeks since the operation and I can't believe I'm going home at last. I feel so much better and I'm looking forward to the next stage of my rehabilitation.

Chapter 3

# Home at Last!

## Day 21 Wednesday 18 August

I awake to the unbelievable sound of rain. Who cares that it's raining on the day I'm going home! My bags are packed and I wait for Garnet to pick me up. I've had my last turn in the pool as an in-patient. As I lie there I think about the wonderful care I've been given in this hospital; the nurses, the food, the physios, all have been first class. How lucky we are to have this facility in our area! I'll be back and I look forward to continuing the treatment in the weeks ahead. I know I need to get back my mobility and strength and coming here will help me achieve that goal.

Writing this diary has also been good for me. When I come to read it I will have forgotten the pain and maybe I'll be shocked at what I've been through. Memories tend to fade but I will have it down in black and white. (As I'm putting this story on my computer it has brought it all back and I realise how much better I am now compared to those early days.)

Garnet picks me up at 10.30am and the joy of walking in the back door of my home is indescribable. It is a freezing cold day with the temperature around 11 degrees. I have to add layers to get warm. Garnet prepares me some toasted sandwiches and a cup of soup which are wonderful. I go back on the hot blanket for a rest after lunch. The warmth on my sore back is bliss. It's still pouring outside. My bed is so comfortable and I feel joyous at being there. There is no place like your own bed in your own home. That night some beautiful flowers are delivered from Justin, welcoming me home. That made me feel good.

## Day 22 Thursday 19 August

Oh, to be in my own bed, on my electric blanket. I had the best night's sleep in ages and Garnet brings me breakfast in bed. I stay there until about 10 o'clock. Being able to wash my hair under the shower makes me feel wonderful. After all, I have been away three weeks and it seems like an eternity.

After lunch I lie down and listen to the radio. I try to do my exercises on the bed and then it's time to get up, sit in my favourite chair and watch more Olympics. I receive phone calls from friends anxious to see how I am. They are pleased I'm up and walking. I ring Justin to thank him for the flowers. It won't be long before he's home on holiday. He and his girlfriend, Karla are coming for a three-week break on 19 November and I can't wait to see them. I hope I'm feeling better by then.

## Day 23 Friday 20 August

I get up early and shower and dress so Garnet can take me to the doctor for a blood test. When I arrive back the tennis girls are here ready to play. It's terrific seeing them. Jan and Bev have come as well. We sit in the sun and discuss how I am progressing while the others go on to play. I enjoy talking to these two girls who have been through the same experience. Eileen Walker arrives with a vase of orchids. They are magnificent. We sit and enjoy a cup of tea together and it's wonderful being out in the open with the sun on my legs. Having the tennis girls around me does wonders for my morale. I am more determined than ever that I will join them on the court as soon as possible. One way or another I will get these bloody knees to move and watching the girls play is just the incentive I need.

By the time they leave I'm tired so I lie down and rest. Tom is coming later to give me a back massage and I'm looking forward to that. My back feels awful and I've decided to have a massage once a week until it feels better. A little pampering is what I need right now.

## Day 24 Saturday 21 August

The guys arrive in the afternoon to play tennis and I go out to watch a few sets. They are pleased to see me walking, albeit on crutches. Garnet's friends have been concerned about me. I enjoy the company and it takes my mind off my woes. My knees are still feeling stiff but I'm not in any pain. I've taken myself off painkillers but I'm still on Warfarin. I'm lucky I didn't get any clots in my legs or lungs as I believe it's common with this type of operation. Being put on Heparin straight away and then Warfarin certainly prevented that complication.

After watching for a while my back gets sore so I go in and lie down. I spend a lot of time lying on my bed as it helps to relieve my back pain.

## Day 25 Sunday 22 August

It's delightful being able to read the Sunday papers over breakfast. Garnet has decided to cook a roast dinner and prepares the vegetables. He has bought a large leg of lamb enough for an army so I imagine we'll be eating it all week. His heart is in the right place. He really is a gem and is going about his jobs cheerfully and is glad to have me home - I think.

I take two walks around the tennis court and later in the afternoon I help Garnet cook the dinner. Mark joins us.

## Day 26 Monday 23 August

Today is my first day of rehab as an out-patient. I awaken feeling dopey having taken two strong painkillers in the night. I really don't want to go but Garnet keeps urging me on. I have to do one hour of exercises and then one hour in the pool. How am I going to manage all that? I'm feeling sick. I want to curl up in bed and stay there but I'm not allowed.

When we arrive at Delmar I plod to the gym, a crutch under each arm, to be warmly greeted by the other patients. Norma is there. I meet Mick, a friend of hers who also has a knee replacement. Anne is a redhead with a bright personality who had her knee done around the same time as I did. Patrick, a Catholic priest, also has a new knee. Josie is our physiotherapist and she takes us through the exercises and I try to do them to the best of my ability. My spirits lift being with these people. We laugh, chat, moan and cry as we put our knees to the ultimate test. How many degrees can you do today?

The bending of the knees is the most painful but essential part of all the exercises. We know how important it is to get them bending but we all hate it. Some are already on the exercise bike but that looks too hard just yet. We move from exercise to exercise and make sure we've done them all before being allowed in the pool. The look of relief is obvious when the hour is up and we all make our way into the warm water.

My two red scars stand out as I painfully make my way into the water. 'You haven't had two done, have you?' I'm asked by other patients who have come only for the pool. Most look incredulous and we exchange stories. I must say it's inspiring talking to others who had knees done before me. I realise I still have a long way to go. Everyone tells me how well I'm going and that makes me feel good. Doing the exercises in the water is certainly much easier than on land. I work as hard as I can and use the soothing water to my advantage. By the time the hour is up I'm exhausted but I still have to join the others for morning tea. This becomes a ritual after our time in the pool and we all look forward to getting together around the table. Cook provides us with a cake or toasted sandwich each time we come. This is all part of the therapy as others join us for that wonderful cup of tea.

As soon as I get home I go and lie down. I don't know what feels worse, my stiff knees or my aching back. I begin to feel sorry for myself. Come on girl, brighten up!

## Day 27 Tuesday 24 August

I am going to the pool only this morning. Robyn rings before I leave. It is good talking to her. She was my writing tutor and she came to Norfolk Island with Catherine and me for the Readers and Writers festival in July. She has a positive outlook on life and is just the one to get me off my backside and cherish another day.

There are only two others in the pool so we have it to ourselves. Mondays are usually crowded with just enough room to walk around but Tuesdays are not so busy. I love my time in the water. Garnet picks me up and as he has a busy day ahead he leaves me to manage on my own. I spend the time sitting in my chair or lying down. I do my exercises and walk around the court a few times. I have to do something to help myself.

Nadia rings to see if she and Cameron can come to see me on Thursday night. They will bring some takeaway. I say yes but instantly regret my decision. I'm usually buggered after my evening meal and don't last long in front of the television. I won't be good company. Why did I say they can come? I will ring back and explain the situation. I'll enjoy seeing them when I'm feeling a bit better.

That evening I go to bed straight after my meal and listen to the radio. 2GB is reporting on the Olympics so I listen for a while before taking a sleeping pill. My nights are generally disturbed. I know it will get better.

## Day 28 Wednesday 25 August

Another visit to the pool does wonders. The afternoon is spent lying on my back. I find the exercises I'm doing for my knees aggravate my back. I'm in a catch 22 situation but the physios keep telling me that exercise is good for it. So why isn't it feeling any better?

I take myself for a walk around the court. My left knee feels heavy and I'm sure I can feel the prosthesis whereas I'm not conscious of it in my right one at all. Funny about that! When I come inside Margaret rings. She is so encouraging. Her knee operation was done over twelve months ago and now she is playing tennis three or four times a week. As she said to me early in the piece, 'I'm not putting my knee in the bottom drawer.' In other words she fully intends to play the game she loves for as long as she can. Life is too short to sit around and do nothing. I admire her attitude. She told me to be kind to myself and not overdo things.

I ring Cameron and suggest they do not come to dinner. I'm just not good company at the moment. There will be time for all that.

## Day 29 Thursday 16 August

Can you believe it? It is exactly one month since the operation. Today I have to be up early to go to rehab by 8am. It's a bit of a rush and I don't feel like going but I know I must. Once I'm with the others I'll be fine. Josie says my knees aren't bending far enough so I will have to work on that. We laugh and joke as we go from exercise to exercise, making sure we don't miss any. I can see Anne trying to make her knees go round on the bike for the first time. It is a struggle but she makes it. I still don't think I'm ready yet. I tell Josie about my bad back and she says it will get better in time. I suppose it has to get used to my new posture. I've been walking in a peculiar way for so long that my back is accustomed to it and now that I have straight legs I must be walking differently. The muscles have to readjust to the new me.

The pool is welcoming after the hard grind and we enjoy ourselves. Today a little Japanese lady arrives with a pained look on her face. I see two scars. No, not another bilateral! When I see her face I realize that must have been how I looked on my first day. I immediately go up to her, sympathize and tell her I have been through the same thing. She is having trouble bending her knees and she looks a picture of misery. My heart goes out to her. I know what she's going through.

When I arrive home I can't wait to lie down. I badly need a rest after the two hours. I'm having another massage this afternoon. I think my back is feeling a little better or is it my imagination? Won't it be wonderful to feel my old self again! This journal has been my way of getting my feelings down on paper. When I look at my cards and flowers I realise how lucky I am to have such good friends. How important they are at a time like this!

## Day 30 Friday 27 August

I had a good night's sleep as I can now turn on my side with a pillow between my legs. Sleeping on my back for all that time was difficult but I managed with the help of pills. I'm about to go to the doctor for another blood test for my Warfarin levels. Surely I'll be able to be taken off it soon! When I arrive back the girls have arrived for tennis. They always cheer me up.

I sit outside to watch the girls play. Our regulars are Peg Baumer, Helena Basden, Faye Rogan and Carolyn Robens. Bev was a regular before her operation as was Nola Munro before her knees began playing up. Margaret has been joining us as well. To see how magically she moves around the court fires me with enthusiasm and gives me hope that I might be able to play like that one day. I look down at my knees and wonder if they will be able to move at all. Of course they will. It's hard to believe at the moment because they feel so heavy and stiff.

To feel the sun on my back and fresh air in my lungs is truly uplifting. I tell myself I can do this but I know I can't be in too big a hurry. Being such an impatient person I want it to happen yesterday. We laugh and joke as we sit and drink our morning tea. They tell me how well I'm doing. Girls, if you only knew!

## Day 31 Saturday 28 August

Hurray! I don't have to go anywhere today. I can stay in bed longer. The guys are coming to play tennis this afternoon. Good, I'll have something to watch and someone to talk to.

## Day 32 Sunday 29 August

While Garnet is doing the shopping after lunch I ask to be dropped off at Mum's. She is living at the Seaside Assisted Living Apartments in Warriewood and I know she is anxious to see me. When I walk down to her unit on my crutches she watches and tells me how well I'm walking. She makes a cup of tea and we sit and chat. By the time Garnet returns my back is really aching and I'm glad to go home. I help Garnet put the groceries away and then go and lie down. My bed is getting a lot of use.

## Day 33 Monday 30 August

Another early start but I like catching up with my fellow patients at rehab. We discuss how we're progressing. I keep telling myself they have only one knee to worry about and I have two! I moan to Josie about my back and she tells me it has a lot to do with posture. I must make sure I sit in an upright chair and not slump.

I see the Japanese lady in the pool again. I can see by her face she's not going too well. It's still hard for her to bend her knees. I try to lift her spirits and tell her it will get better. That is what rehab is all about, giving each other support.

## Day 34 Tuesday 31 August

I made a big step forward today. I manage to sit downstairs and help Garnet with his end of month statements. Garnet has his own Real Estate business which he runs from home and I'm his offsider but while I've been laid up he's had to manage on his own. Now it is time for me to help out and I am proud that I last the whole morning. I sit propped up in a chair and having something to do is good for me. It takes my mind off myself for a while.

I'm feeling more hopeful now. Tomorrow I'm going to do my Creative Memories which is putting photos in albums creatively. I've been doing it for a while and have done albums for my three boys and one for my brother David for his 60th birthday. I am in the process of doing an album for me. Hopefully once I'm immersed in that I won't notice my aching back and painful knees.

## Day 35 Wednesday 1 September

When I get up my knees are really stiff. I had been in bed since 7.30pm the night before. Thankfully I'm going to the pool today.

That will help I'm sure. As usual the water does its magic. I come out feeling much better. I even manage four times around the court when I return home. I'm still using one crutch.

Catherine comes to visit in the afternoon and we sit in the outside cabana and enjoy a cup of tea. She has just been to the Mall shopping. When will I be able to do things like that? The day is cold but the sun warms us up. Catherine and I discuss our writing and other things. She has given me wonderful support. I really enjoy her visits.

## Day 36 Thursday 2 September

I do well at the gym today but still my left knee isn't as good as my right when Josie measures it. I ask if I can have it measured again after being in the pool and she agrees. She also asks if I would like to come an extra day and I say yes. Next week I'll be coming on Monday, Wednesday and Thursday mornings. Surely I will get better quicker with all that extra exercise. Off we go for our hour in the pool. I see Michael and we compare notes. I'm jealous at how well he's doing but I mustn't be impatient. I go back for another measure and sure enough my knees are bending better after being in the water. I feel pleased.

Morning tea is fun and it's good to sit around and listen to the others. We are all at different stages and it's encouraging to see how they're progressing. I suppose I am as well.

I walk around the court five times when I arrive home. Soon I'll be able to throw the crutch away. Then I'll know I'm on the road to recovery.

## Day 37 Friday 3 September

It is great seeing the tennis girls again. Talking to them takes me my mind off my sore back. Rain interrupts play so we have our cup of tea in the meantime. Luckily it eases off and the girls play another set. Oh, to be out there with them!

In the afternoon I sit at my computer working on my Broken Hill story and I am amazed being able to sit for so long with my knees under the desk. Once I'm in my imaginary world I forget all my troubles and the time ticks by. Tom comes to give me another back massage. Heaven!

## Day 38 Saturday 4 September

I enjoy being able to sleep in this morning and get up a little later than usual. Garnet goes off to show some flats while I potter around the house. I do my exercises and some laps around the court. You can't say I'm not trying.

I watch the guys play tennis in the afternoon for a while and then work on my computer. Cameron comes to pick up Garnet later in the afternoon as they are going to Rat Park for the union match as a treat for Fathers' Day. I speak to Justin in Florida and he tells me he is waiting for the hurricane that is due any time. Luckily for them they have shutters around the outside of their house. They just have to wait patiently until it blows over. I tell him to ring me the next day if the phone lines are still intact to say they are safe. (They were fine with no damage, thank goodness but it must have been very frightening all the same.)

## Day 39 Sunday 5 September

I have a quiet day with no visitors. I work on my novel and then read my book. I can't believe it's time for my first check up tomorrow. Doesn't time fly when you're having fun?

Chapter 4

# At the Six Week Mark!

## Day 40 Monday 6 September

This is a big day as I'm seeing Dr William L Walter, the son of my doctor at his Dee Why surgery. He is also an orthopedic surgeon and they assist each other. I am going to rehab first and then Garnet will take me to his rooms. I arrive early so I sit and read. When the doctor calls me in I triumphantly walk into his surgery holding one crutch in the air. He is tall and handsome, almost film star material.

'See, I don't need it,' I smile. The doctor tells me to get up on the table so he can examine me. I have to bend both knees and he notices the angle of each. I tell him that my right knee is much better than my left and ask him why. He explains that the two knees were not done the same as they each had different problems and that could be the reason they don't feel the same.

'More exercise needed. Keep working at it,' Dr Walter tells me. I'm told I don't have to wear the dreaded white stockings. Hallelujah! I can also give the Warfarin away. That is good news. I almost skip out of his surgery. As I'm walking to the car I realise I've forgotten to ask when I can drive. Back I go and ask his secretary. She says I can drive at six weeks which is only a few days away but that I should have a practice first. I intend to do that. I can also give away the crutches. What a big day this turns out to be! I must be at the turning point but how wrong can you be!

## Day 41 Tuesday 7 September

I can't believe we're into September. The year is rushing past. Mum comes up to see me in the afternoon and we watch the US Open together. My back holds up for the two hours. What an improvement!

## Day 42 Wednesday 8 September

After my hour in the gym and another hour in the pool Garnet drops me off at my hairdresser's home to get my hair permed. I am thrilled I last the three hours that it takes to transform me. It makes me feel like a new person. I'm beginning to feel like my old self again.

## Day 43 Thursday 9 September

It's now six weeks since the operation. It's hard to believe. I meet an Indian lady in the pool today and she had one knee done two weeks ago. Poor thing, she can't bend it so today she is going to be put under anesthetic to have it bent by the doctor. She is not looking forward to the procedure. I'll be interested to see how it goes for her.

The Japanese lady is not happy. She's still having trouble bending her knees. She thinks she's going home today. Her son came out from Japan to look after her husband who unfortunately had to be put into a nursing home because of dementia. The poor lady has no one to go home to, as her son is flying out today. Shame he couldn't stay another week or two but I suppose business calls. My heart goes out to her.

My knees bend quite well today with 115 degrees in my right and 110 in my left and that's before I go in the water. Tom comes in the afternoon and gives me a leg and back massage. I'm so lucky to be able to have that done. I'm sure it's aiding my progress.

## Day 44 Friday 10 September

A big day today! I drove my car for the first time since the operation. Garnet came with me and made me do lots of stops and starts. I felt like a beginner again. He even made me do a hill start. I found it difficult getting my left foot across to the brake but somehow I managed. My car is an automatic, thank goodness. Now I'll be able to drive myself to rehab without having to rely on my husband.

The girls didn't come to tennis today so I busy myself in the office doing a few jobs. I print off a copy of my Broken Hill story for my writing friend Joan to edit for me. I am making big strides forward.

## Day 45 Saturday 11 September

Life is getting back to normal although I'm still not up to showing flats for Garnet. Maybe next week. The US Open is on television so I sit and watch. After a while I go outside and watch the guys run around the tennis court. They take it so seriously. No holds barred. Some get frustrated when the shots they played 20 years ago don't come off. I can't wait to play again. I join the fellows for a drink afterwards and enjoy the camaraderie.

I'm still not able to sit for long periods so I lie down and read a lot. I suppose this is all part of recuperating. Reading is good for my writing so I should be grateful to have this time to read lots of books. Usually, I'm so busy that reading takes a back seat.

## Day 46 Sunday 12 September

It's blowing a gale today. In the night I got up to record Leyton Hewitt's final so I can watch it with Mum today. When I ring her to tell her the time I'll be picking her up, she blurts out who won. Blast! I like to watch a match without knowing the result. Too late now. It isn't quite the same knowing who had won but we enjoy watching anyway. Garnet goes to visit his mother who hasn't been well.

I drive Mum back home and feel quite confident. Knowing that I can take myself to rehab tomorrow is a great feeling. They say around six weeks you start feeling normal and I suppose that's right. Just think how good I'll be in another six weeks! Maybe my left knee will begin feeling like my right. Maybe? (Maybe not!)

## Day 47 Monday 13 September

I drive myself to rehab but I think I may have overdone the exercises as I'm suffering in the back area. I must remember to take things slowly. My right leg was 113 degrees and my left was 105. I wonder if the left will ever catch up.

## Day 48 Tuesday 14 September

It is Cameron's birthday today so I ring before he goes to work. Garnet is going out with Mark and Cameron tonight for a beer tasting and I will be on my own. That's all right. I'm quite happy being by myself. The thought of going out at night is a long way off. I go to see my Bunka (Japanese Embroidery) ladies in the morning. Bunka is an enjoyable craft. I've been doing it for a few years and have done some lovely pictures which adorn my walls and those of my children. A picture is printed onto fabric and attached to a wooden frame. We punch coloured threads with a long needle to make the picture and then it gets framed. Jenny, our tutor usually takes them to her framer and he does a great job. The outcome is always fantastic. I haven't seen a dud yet. When I arrive the room is packed with cheerful women, all chattering while they work.

I stay for half an hour and then go for a walk along Narrabeen Lakes. It has been a long time since I've walked along these peaceful shores. It is a calm, sunny day and not too cold. I take one crutch with me and go slowly down the path. I don't go too far as I get tired so I sit on a bench on the way back and watch the ducks. It is wonderful soaking up the sun.

## Day 49 Wednesday 15 September

I work hard in the gym today and my knee-bends measure 113 and 110. The left one is catching up. Go, you good thing! The time in the pool is enjoyable, chatting to others who come week after week trying to get their hip, leg or back better. The Indian lady who had her knee manipulated came to the pool today with a pained look on her face. Her knee is only bending to 80 degrees and she is trying everything to get it to bend further. I feel sorry for her and try to give her some encouragement. I wonder how she is doing now.

Morning tea is fun as we wait to see what delicious surprise cook has baked for us. I go for a walk around the lake on my way home. I'm still using one crutch for safety purposes. I'm lucky to have many beautiful places to walk in my district. I like walking on the flat and around Narrabeen Lakes is perfect.

My friend Jocelyn comes to visit in the afternoon and we catch up on all the news. She brought a delicious bun and we have a cup of tea to go with it. That night I watch television until 8.30pm. I bring my straight backed computer chair to sit in. When I decide to get up, it runs away from me and I crash to the floor. Not a pretty sight! Luckily Garnet is there to pick me up. I feel such a fool and no harm is done. However, at this stage of my rehabilitation I could have done without that.

## Day 50 Thursday 16 September

It is seven weeks since the operation. Can you imagine it? I can now go up and down stairs, drive a car, walk long distances, bend my knees so I'm not doing too badly. The physio says I'm walking well. It's wonderful having two straight legs. I'm sure I'm a lot taller. I can wear shorts again. I try to jog in the water today. Lifting my legs is quite difficult and a strange feeling. Norma has only one more week of rehab while I have two but I have extra times in the pool which I will definitely use.

It's a beautiful day and it's getting warmer. I feel good. My back is settling down at last.

## Day 51 Friday 17 September

What an enjoyable morning it was! We have six for tennis and our traveller Peg has returned once more. Margaret comes as well. We are always pleased to see her. Bev and Norma come for a chat. We decide that it is amazing that there are now four of us with new knees, five if we count Jan who has decided not to play again. I am definitely going to be President of this exclusive club, 'The New Knees Club.' I know Bev and Norma will be playing before me but I will get there sooner or later. I am determined.

It is great talking to the girls, comparing our knees and how they feel at this point. Bev is quite a few months ahead of Norma and me. Margaret is a long way ahead of all of us. We all envy how she can run around the court. After the girls leave I walk around the court six times. Come on Pam, get those knees moving and you can play too.

## Day 52 Saturday 18 September

I actually put my real estate hat on today and open a flat for Garnet in Chatswood. I must admit I'm glad it was only open for half an hour. By the time I drive home my back is really sore so I lie down for a while. I am going to my FAW (Fellowship of Australian Writers) meeting and I'm being picked up by Catherine. I take my pillow and hot bottle. Thank goodness I did, as the heat helps me get through the meeting. I get up a couple of times and walk around the table. I'm pleased to last the distance.

Sleeping at night is becoming a problem. I take half a sleeping tablet but for the last two nights it hasn't got me off to sleep and I've had to get up and take the other half. What's going on? I toss and turn keeping Garnet awake.

## Day 53 Sunday 19 September

A big test today. We're having visitors. It's the family and I have to prepare the salads and get through the whole day. Can I do it? It turns out to be a strange day - rain in the morning, sunshine in the afternoon and a storm at night. I manage quite well but I'm tired by the time they all leave. I feel elated that I've been able to entertain guests and not have to go and lie down in the middle. I must be improving.

## Day 54 Monday 20 September

In the afternoon Garnet takes me shopping with him. This is my first time since the operation and it's a strange experience. Garnet watches over me like a mother hen, not allowing his chick too much leeway. I know he does it because he cares and doesn't want me to fall flat on my face in front of shoppers. I manage to stay on my feet and not disgrace myself. Pushing the trolley helps me get around the aisles. Garnet brings the groceries inside while I help put things away. Surely I'll be able to do it on my own soon.

## Day 55 Tuesday 21 September

What a big day I've had today! In the morning I went to Bunka with my pillow and hot bottle. I lasted the two hours quite well with a walk in between. I then headed towards Bayview for a re-union with my writing group. This is the first time since the operation that I've been able to join them. It is at Mary's house and it is fun catching up with the ladies. They can't get over my straight legs and how well I am walking and how much taller I now am. That made me feel good. As we sit and eat lunch we chat and enjoy each other's company. It is a convivial group and we always have lots to talk about.

We then read our pieces of work. We listen and make comments afterwards. We try to encourage each other with our writing. We have been meeting ever since completing writing classes with Robyn McWilliam at the Manly Warringah Community College at Narrabeen about four years ago. There is Catherine who is working on children's stories and is in the process of publishing a picture book for young children. Her daughter-in-law is doing the illustrations. I can't wait to see it. (I've now seen it and it's fabulous.) Mary has already published a children's story and illustrated it herself and is working on another book. She is a fine artist and painted the front cover for my autobiography. Joan has a wonderful way with words and I have entrusted her to edit my last two books and I'm going to ask her to do my Broken Hill story. She is involved with netball training and is an ex-teacher. I enjoy listening to her pieces of work. Jenny has a wonderful sense of humour which shows in her writing. We have enjoyed many of her funny stories. She is in the process of writing her life story. The going is tough for Jenny but I hope she makes it. Marjorie has not been in the best of health and hasn't had time to write as much as she would like. Her work is always of a high standard. Bea is writing a biography of an important sculptor in her family and has done a great deal of research for this story.

All in all it has been beneficial for all of us to come together and inspire each other. I left that day about 3pm, pleased that I was able to enjoy normal activities again.

## Day 56 Wednesday 22 September

It is nearly eight weeks - the time has flown since I've been home. Only one more week of rehab. The physio told me today that in two weeks I can have a hit of tennis. I nearly fell through the floor. Boy! I thought I had a long way to go. She said to just stand there and hit the ball - that's what I was doing before the operation with my gammy leg - I can't wait.

## Day 57 Thursday 23rd September

There were not many in the pool today and that was good. I still have seven pool visits to go and that's comforting. I arrange with Norma and Bev to come next week to have a hit on the court. We've got to start sometime and why not now. We're all nervous and wonder if we'll be able to move at all but we're cracking our necks to play again. Psychologically it will be good for us.

## Day 58 Friday 24th September

It rained today so no tennis. I was disappointed as I enjoy seeing the girls. I ring Mum and take her to lunch instead. Later in the afternoon I take myself for a walk around the tennis court and decide to jog. I find I can do it so I alternate the walking with the jogging. I then stand on the court and pretend to hit a forehand and backhand. I then move forwards and backwards and side to side.

Tears come to my eyes. 'I can do it,' I keep telling myself. Back to running and walking and down at the other end I practise my service action. By this time I'm getting quite emotional. Tears begin falling down my cheeks as I realize I am going to be able to play again. Without my crutch I have much more freedom to move. I feel quite ecstatic. I'm going to ask Garnet to give me a hit on Sunday, I promise myself. Bring it on!

## Day 59 Saturday 25 September

I work for Garnet today and even receive an application for a flat that has been hard to let. I do hope it goes ahead. At night Garnet takes me out to dinner at our favourite Italian restaurant in Narrabeen. This is my first meal out since the operation and I savour every mouthful. I take my cushion and hot water bottle. How much longer do I have to be attached to them?

## Day 60 Sunday 26 September

As promised, Garnet gives me a hit of tennis. I stroke the ball quite well but I can't run very far. That will come in time. I practise my serve and to my surprise I find the service box many times. I feel jubilant coming off the court but realise I still have a way to go before joining my friends. Oh well, I have to start somewhere. Now I can only go forward positively.

## Day 61 Monday 27 September

Hurrah, my last week of rehab! I take along a story I have written called "The Pool" about my time in Delmar and give a copy to Anne, the fiery redhead, to Norma and to Josie, the physio. After my session in the pool I go to the Mall and buy myself a pair of new tennis shoes at Rebel Sports. I'm deadly serious about playing again and I think I deserve new shoes. I've had my other ones for ages and they are thoroughly worn out.

I take Mum shopping in the afternoon, the first time without Garnet. I come home very proud of myself.

## Day 62 Tuesday 28 September

I find out at Bunka that two of our girls are going in to hospital next week, one to have a new hip and the other a new knee. I'm able to give them some advice. Poor things! They're not young ladies but I'm sure they will go well. Both are going to Delmar for rehab. Maybe I'll see them when I go to the pool for my extra visits.

## Day 63 Wednesday 29 September

Second last gym session. I will miss the fun times we've had over the last six weeks. It has done wonders for me. Being able to air my grievances and have a good moan has been good. I hope I don't go backwards on my own. I know I must keep exercising.

Oh no, it begins to rain after lunch! This is the day Norma and Bev are coming to have a hit on the court. I keep looking at the weather and it doesn't look like stopping. I tell the girls to come and we'll have a cup of tea and it may stop enough for us to get on the court later. The rain does stop and out we go, eager to hit the ball. At first the balls spray everywhere. No one can hit directly to the other person. We laugh and keep trying. By the end of the session we're doing a lot better. We even practise our serves but it is difficult to run for balls out of reach.

At the end we all feel fantastic. We have taken the first step to playing again. Being out there with the girls was joy enough for me.

## Day 64 Thursday 30 September

Nine weeks today! This is my last rehab session. Delmar has done wonders for my recovery. Where has the time gone? My left knee is bending to 110 degrees and my right 116. Not too bad! I have to do my walking test. On the first day we were given a short distance to cover and it was timed. We now have to do it again to see how much quicker we've become. I do it in 5.3 seconds. Pretty damn good!! I must admit I cheated and ran the distance when I should have walked. My first time on crutches had been slow and torturous. I have come a long way although my left knee doesn't feel wonderful. I wish it was like my right one. Will it ever feel normal or will it always feel like there's a foreign object restricting my movement? Perhaps I should go and see the surgeon for confirmation that it's all right.

Now I'm on my own. No more being told to bend that knee, lift that leg, ride the bike and smile! We tried to smile but it was hard at times. Being with others kept you on your toes and made you do things you hated doing because the others were doing it so why couldn't you? I'll now have to be disciplined to continue doing them on my own. Can I do it? You do want to play tennis again, don't you? Of course, so get on your bike and ride!

Chapter 5

# Back to Normality

## Day 65 Friday 1 October

Tennis is called off - it is pouring. It's wonderful to see the rain. I have a lazy day but I did ring to make an appointment to see the doctor about my left knee next Wednesday. I'm going for my peace of mind. No good worrying that something may be wrong. Better to find out now than later. Hurrah, Tom is coming tonight. My back is still not good. Garnet is bringing home Chinese.

## Day 66 Saturday 2 October

The guys come to play tennis and I go and watch them later in the afternoon. Bev Lambley, one of the player's wives comes out to see me and shares our drinks and nibbles. It is good to see her.

## Day 67 Sunday 3 October

Garnet and I go for a walk around Narrabeen Lakes in the morning. It is a beautiful place to walk. I love watching the ducks and I see some children feeding them. There are canoes on the lake and they make a pretty sight. In the afternoon I take Mum to the movies to see Wimbledon and we quite enjoy it. I go with my pillow and hot water bottle. How I wish I could discard them! Hopefully soon.

## Day 68 Monday 4 October

I go shopping by myself and I put all the food away and then work on the computer. It is a beautiful sunny day.

## Day 69 Tuesday 5 October

I go to the rehab pool and enjoy doing all the exercises in the warm water. My left knee is still a bother.

## Day 70 Wednesday 6 October

After a session in the pool I attend my appointment with the doctor. To my surprise, Margaret is already sitting in the waiting room.

'What are you doing here?' I ask her.

'I've come to be with you,' she replies. What a lovely thing to do, I thought. She is a kind girl and has given me so much support. After sitting in the waiting room for a while the receptionist announces that the doctor has been delayed and won't be in for at least another hour. I was all for cancelling and making another appointment, but Margaret said no.

'I'll stay with you. It doesn't matter I have nothing else to do. You must find out about your knee. Come on, we'll go and have a cup of coffee.' I speak to the receptionist on the way out and say we'll be back in a while. We find a little coffee shop and sit at the outside tables and chat. Shoppers hurry past and the time slips by. I'm glad for Margaret's company. Back we go to the waiting room until at last I'm called in. The doctor tests both knees and it is obvious my right moves and bends better than my left. He then tells me I'm to have both knees X-rayed as well as my hips and a bone scan.

I imagine my doctor is being super careful as he says there's a minimal chance of anything being wrong. I suppose I'm a little disappointed that I have to do all that. I was hoping he was going to say there was nothing wrong and just get on with it. I tell Margaret and she's pleased he is being thorough and it will be good for my peace of mind to know one way or the other. I say goodbye and thank her for sticking it out with me. I really appreciated her being there. She has been with me the whole journey from my first visit to this important check up. Thanks Margaret!

I ring Mum when I get home and she's disappointed. I suspect she thought the doctor was going to say there was nothing wrong, but he can't see through skin, can he? I did go to him with a complaint so if he had dismissed me offhandedly I would have been dissatisfied. This way I'll have an answer. I have to go back to see him in a month.

## Day 71 Thursday 7 October

Ten weeks today. I have a quiet day and must admit I'm feeling a bit sorry for myself.

## Day 72 Friday 8 October

As I look out the window I see that it's going to be a fine day. Good, the girls can play today. I need their cheerful company. Bev and Norma are coming to hit with each other. I have decided to leave playing until I see the doctor again. Maybe I rushed in a bit too soon. The girls arrive and begin playing. I talk to Bev and Norma about how I'm feeling. Bev tells me not to be so impatient and that everything will be fine. She is now seven months down the track and is feeling good. I watch when she hits with Norma and see that they're moving well on the court. Good for them! I wish it was me!

## Day 73 Saturday 9 October

I open two flats for inspection and feel quite sick at the second one. My head is spinning and I hope I can make it home. I'm thankful to get home and lie down. I go down later to have a drink with the guys and then watch the election results unfold. John Howard is returned with an increased majority.

## Day 74 Sunday 10 October

I feel quite dizzy and sick all day. I don't do anything. What's wrong with me?

## Day 75 Monday 11 October

I go to the rehab pool and see my Bunka friend Inge who has had one knee replaced. She tells me she had it done under an epidural only and could hear the chain saw. How dreadful! Thank goodness I was out cold. She had it done that way because of her heart problems but she did not enjoy the experience. Bless her, after all she is 79. She looks good. I go around to see Carol but she has already gone home. She only had a hip replaced! I rest all afternoon. I'm sick of feeling this way. I must pick up soon.

## Day 76 Tuesday 12 October

I see my own doctor for a blood test. I decide to go to Bunka to cheer myself up but I feel lousy and one of the ladies drives me home. Garnet comes back with her and picks up my car. I'm feeling lightheaded and dizzy. I spend the afternoon lying down. It's a hot day so I have my fan going. I decide to venture into our pool but it's freezing. I go in inch by inch. So different to Delmar's heated pool. I persevere and try to do some exercises and I must admit I feel good afterwards. The cold water is wonderful for my knees.

## Day 77 Wednesday 13 October

I go in our pool again early in the morning and the water is still COLD. It's invigorating and after my shower I feel good. I go around to find out the results of my blood test and everything is OK. The doctor thinks I may have had a virus that's going around. He gives me some Stemital for the dizziness. The day is getting hotter; 38-40 degrees! The water in the pool is still cold but refreshing in the afternoon. Margaret rings and cheers me up as always and I tell her my back is feeling better.

## Day 78 Thursday 14 October

It's 11 weeks since the operation. Time marches on. More exercises in the pool. At least I'm doing something to help myself. I must do this every day.

## Day 79 Friday 15 October

I arise early to go in our pool and the temperature outside is quite cool so the water feels quite bearable. I enjoy doing the exercises and even do a few laps on my back. I feel good when I come out. The girls come for tennis and Bev plays her first set with the others. She goes very well. I'm jealous but my time will come. I'm not ready yet and I know it.

In the afternoon Garnet and I go down to the bike shop in Dee Why to hire an exercise bike. Unfortunately, the one they hire out isn't big enough for my long legs. We end up buying a more expensive one. Will it get used? Will we get our money's worth? Time will tell. I know when I tried it out in the shop my back felt sore, so I'll have to be careful I don't overdo it.

Tom comes in the evening and tells me to go slowly and record my time and distance each day when I get on the bike. Build up gradually, he says. I will take his advice.

## Day 80 Saturday 16 October

I feel better than last Saturday and manage to do my two open houses quite successfully although I don't see many people. Catherine picks me up after lunch to take me to Forest FAW (Fellowship of Australian Writers) and we have an enjoyable meeting.

## Day 81 Sunday 17 October

Garnet sets off to do the lawns at his mother's house. I enthusiastically do some jobs around our place. I feel good doing them. By the afternoon I'm feeling tired but still manage to take Mum shopping. I put all the food away and do some ironing. I have a busy week ahead of me. I hope I can get through it.

## Day 82 Monday 18 October

I'm glad I'm going to the rehab pool this morning because it's cold outside and raining. The warm water is wonderful after my cold pool but I know my time coming here is nearly over. Later in the morning I go for lunch with two teacher friends Barbara and Lesley at Buddha Belly on Mona Vale Road. It is so cold as the place is only protected by plastic sheeting and there is plenty of room for the wind to swirl around. I didn't dress appropriately and I shivered through the meal. After we finished our lunch I invited the girls back to my place for a cup of tea. I couldn't wait to put on a warm jumper. I had taught with Barbara and Lesley at Dee Why Primary School in the late 60s and Barbara and I have remained close friends ever since. It was nice catching up and reminiscing about old times. After they leave I prepare dinner as Cameron and Nadia are coming. It will be great to see them.

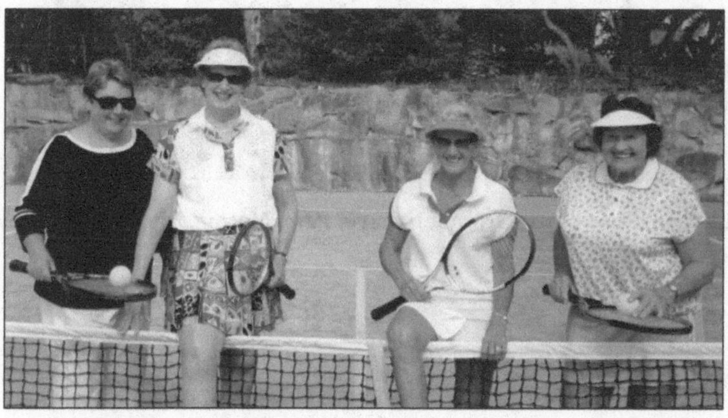

**The New Knees Club - from left: Jan (2 knees), Pam (2 knees), Margaret (1 knee), Bev (1 knee). Norma was missing that day.**

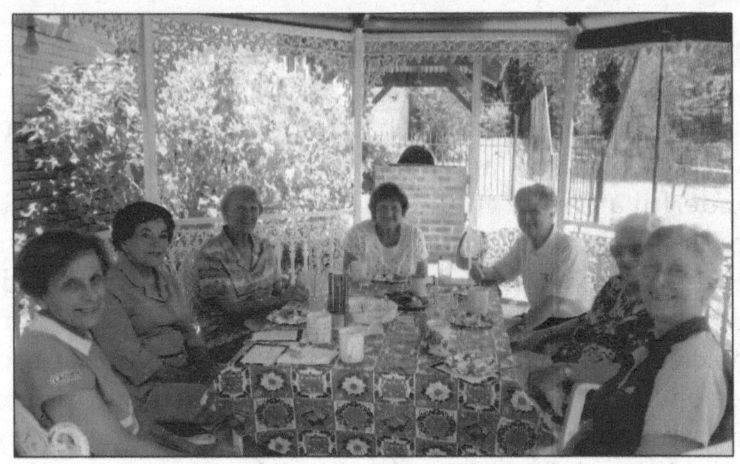

**At our Christmas party - from left: Peg, Eileen, Thelma, Bev, Helena, Brenda (my Mum), Carolyn.**

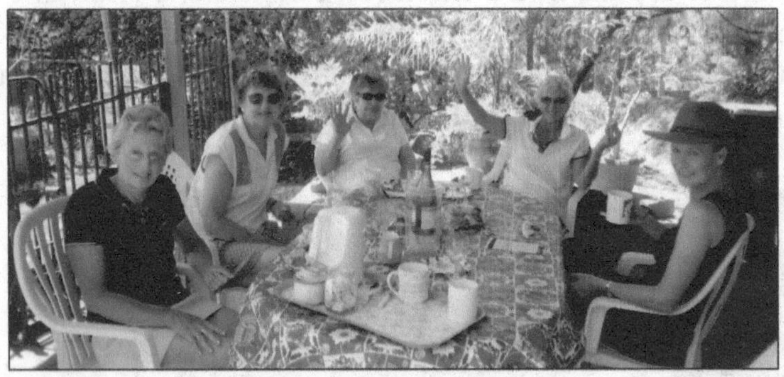

**At the Christmas party - from left: Faye, Pam, Norma, Margaret and Sue.**

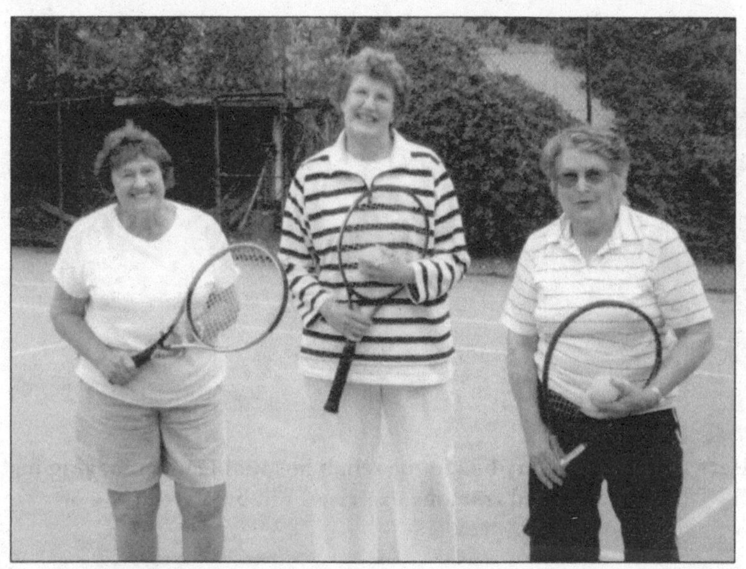

**Our first hit - from left: Bev, Pam and Norma. What a joyful day!**

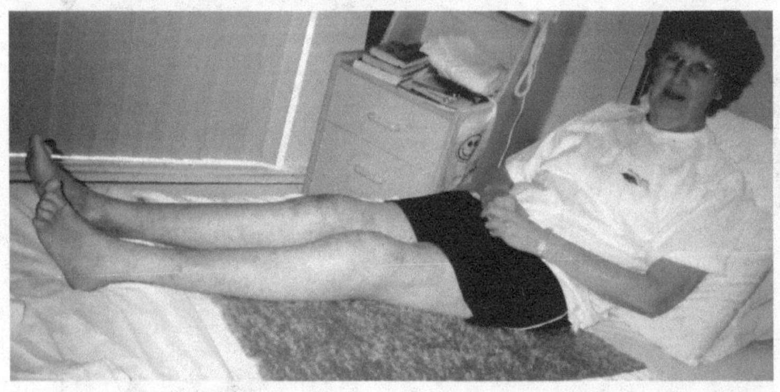

**Here I am lying on my bed in the rehab hospital Delmar, having just returned from my exercises. I'm buggered!**

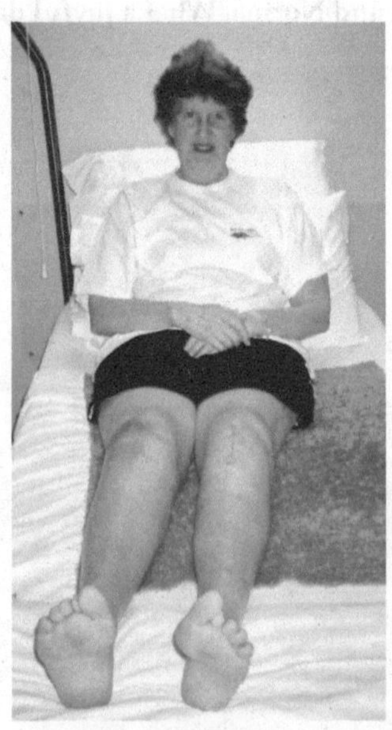

**A good view of my scars! Poor me!**

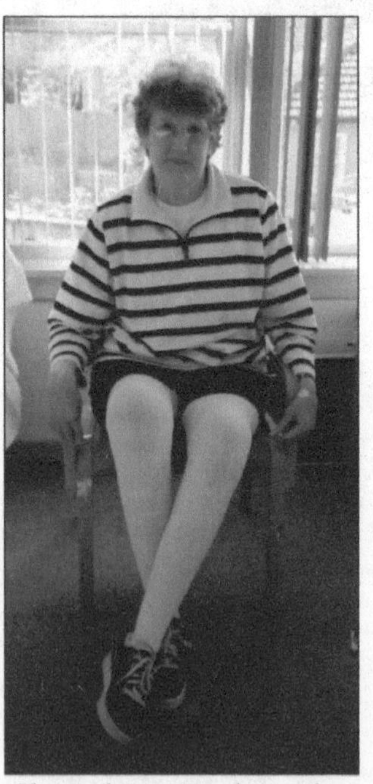

**I'm trying to push one knee as far back as I can with the other leg. This one hurts. I have a roller blade under my left foot to make it go back further.**

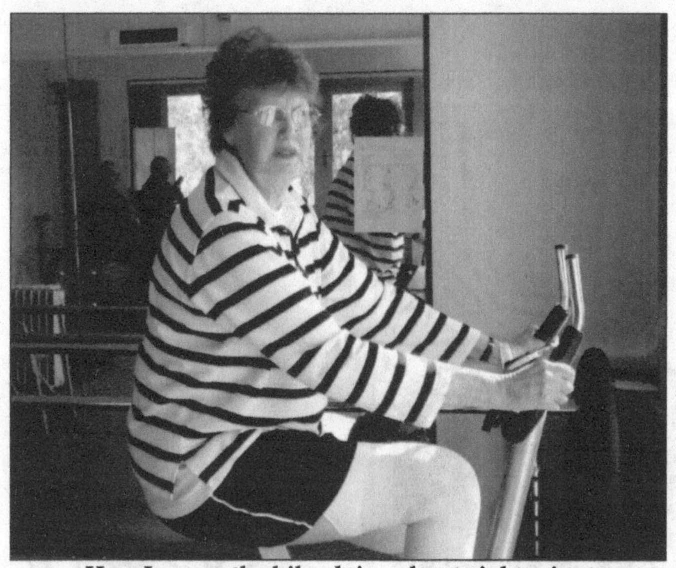

**Here I am on the bike doing about eight minutes.**

**Don't the white stockings look attractive?**

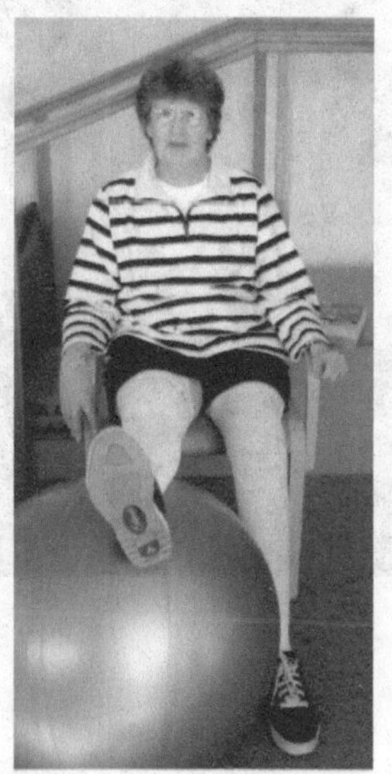

**I didn't mind this exercise. It was for straightening the leg.**

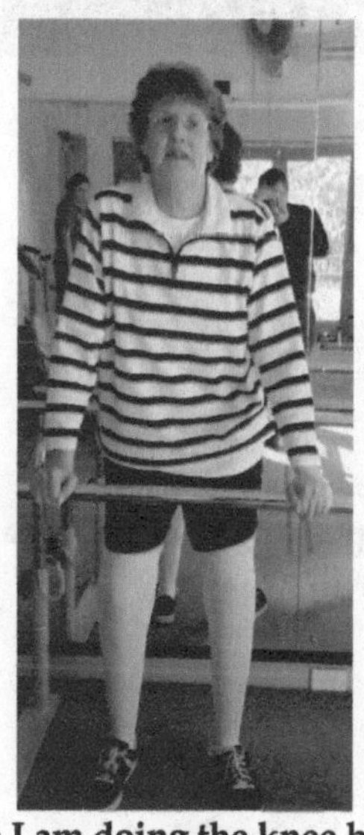

**Here I am doing the knee bends at the bar.**
**This hurt!**

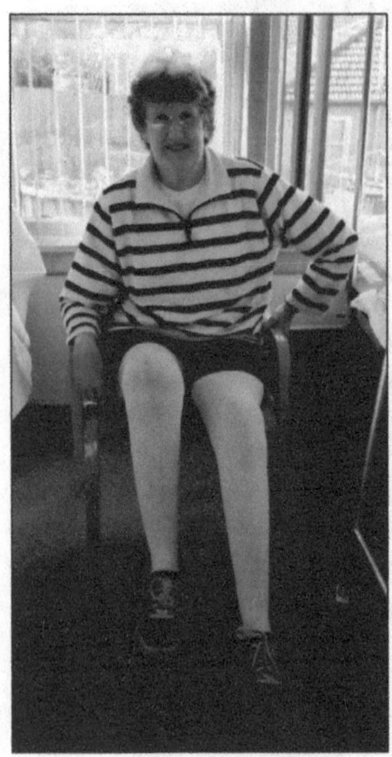

**I am using a roller blade to make my knees bend.**

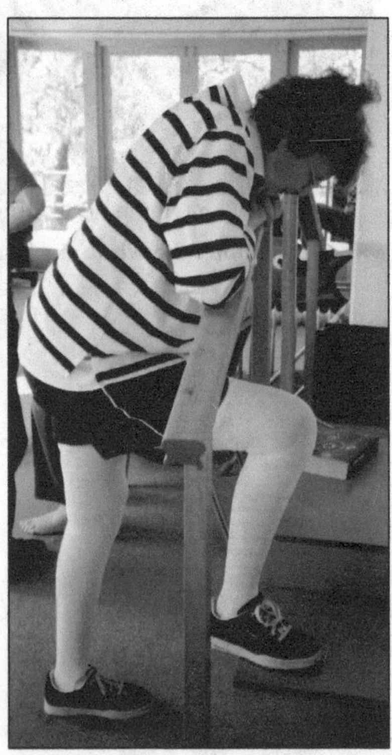

**I hated this exercise.
I am pushing my knee as far as it will go.**

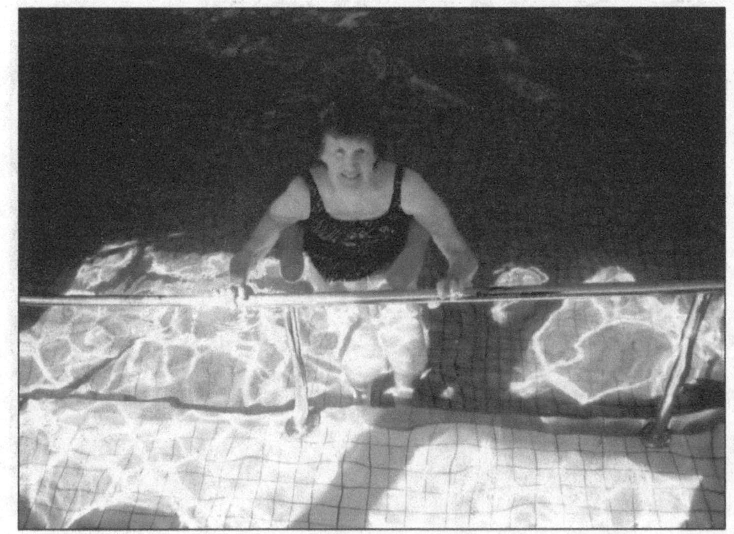

**Here I am with a red floatie under my arms for support, trying to bend my knees. It was so enjoyable in the warm water.**

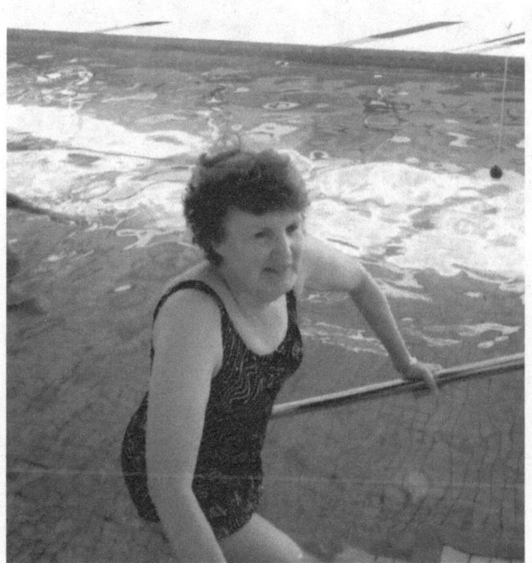

**Getting up the steps was a big effort.**

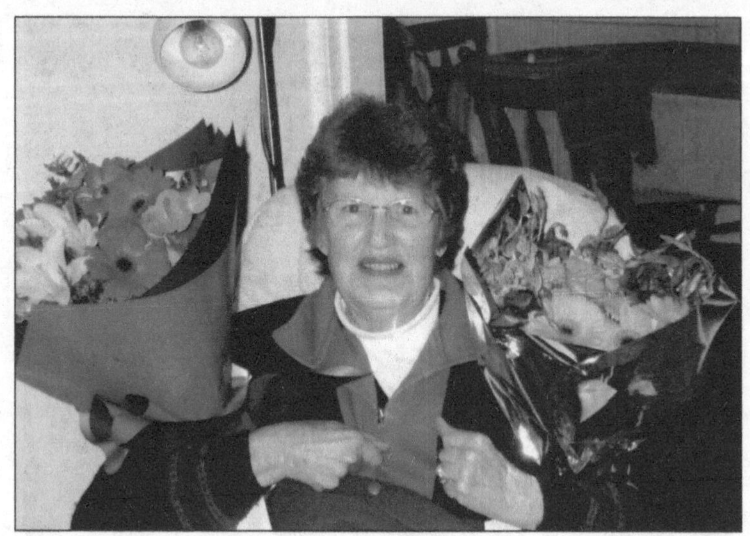

**Home at last!**
**Two beautiful bunches of flowers were waiting for me.**
**It was such a joy to be home.**

Chapter 6

# At the Three Month Mark!

## Day 85 Thursday 21 October

It's now three months since the operation. I wish I could rejoice but my left knee won't let me. Perhaps it's all in my imagination and everyone goes through the same anguish. I wish I knew. (Now would have been a good time to put my piece in the Insearch column and find out if others were suffering like me!) I decide to go to the rehab pool as it's a wet miserable day. It pelted down during the night. I only have two more sessions so my pool at home had better heat up. With all the rain it's probably freezing cold.

I lie back in the water and enjoy the warmth and then do my exercises. I love coming here. I give my knees a good workout and swear at my left one and tell it to hurry up and feel normal. After lunch I work on the computer typing my story about the operation. It's good being able to sit at the computer without too much discomfort and it's interesting to read just what I went through those first few weeks. I have to admit how much better I am now.

## Day 86 Friday 22 October

Rain, rain and more rain! No tennis today. I potter around the house and help Garnet downstairs.

## Day 87 Saturday 23 October

A normal Saturday - show flats in the morning and prepare sweets for visitors who are coming for a BBQ on Sunday. Garnet takes me to the local Chinese restaurant at night.

## Day 88 Sunday 24 October

We have our very good friends the Obermanns for lunch. Barbara and Bruce are our dearest friends and we go back a long way. We always enjoy their company. The day is dull and overcast. Luckily we get through the cooking before the rain begins and then retire to eat indoors. It was a full on day but I came through remarkably well. By evening my back is sore so I don't stay up too late.

## Day 89 Monday 25 October

This is my second last time in the rehab pool. I work hard and come out feeling good. I do some shopping in the afternoon and arrive home tired. My left knee still feels uncomfortable. If the X-rays say there is nothing wrong I'll just have to get used to it. It may come good in time. To make matters worse the exercise bike has broken down. The pedals won't go round without grating; just as I'm building up my time and strength. Garnet will have to take it back to the shop for them to take a look. What a nuisance!

## Day 90 Tuesday 26 October

I attend my Bunka group in the morning and my writing group in the afternoon. It is an enjoyable day and my back holds up well. What a relief!

## Day 91 Wednesday 27 October

Garnet and I attend a three hour Real Estate course at the Harbord Diggers in the afternoon. The chair is most uncomfortable but I get through it reasonably well.

## Day 92 Thursday 28 October

I decide to go to Warringah Mall to do some Christmas shopping. I had forgotten how far you have to walk and by the end of two hours I'm exhausted. I run into my friend Jan and her daughter Nicole and I have a moan to them. Jan sympathises as she understands only too well what I'm going through. I find a seat and sit down with what I have already bought. I've done enough for one day. Time to go home. My legs are feeling tight and it's not easy walking. When I arrive home I make the comment to Garnet that I wish I had my old knees back and he says, 'No, you don't,' very emphatically. At this point of time I don't like my new ones very much.

## Day 94 Friday 29 October

I should be over the worst by now and feeling great but I'm not. Someone has been telling porkies. I help Garnet with his end of month statements while the girls play tennis. I join them for a cup of tea later. Oh, to be able to run around like them! What a joy when I can play again! When will that ever happen? Maybe never? I can't and won't believe that!

## Day 94 Saturday 30 October

A usual Saturday, inspections in the morning and work on the computer in the afternoon. Thank goodness I love writing as it certainly fills in the hours. My computer room is my haven. I forget everything when I'm sitting in front of my best friend. Well, not perhaps everything as I am writing about my bilateral!

## Day 96 Sunday 31 October

Early in the morning I go for a walk around the lake but it is an effort. My left knee is not feeling good. Am I imagining it or is there really something wrong? Please let me find out soon! I take Mum to the movies and we see *Shall We Dance* which is most enjoyable. My friend Bronwen comes with us. It is good to see her. She has just been on a wonderful trip around Western Australia. It was interesting to hear all about it.

## Day 97 Monday 1 November

I'm sad. It is my last day in the rehab pool. I have really enjoyed coming here. It has helped with my feeling of well being and rehabilitation. I'm going to miss meeting the people and of course the heavenly warm water. I may pay for some extra sessions. I'll wait and see. My own pool may be warm enough soon. In the afternoon Garnet takes the broken bike back to the shop at last and returns with a new one. I do two five minute sessions. My knees feel all right doing it. I wish they didn't feel so stiff when I stop but I can't exercise all day.

## Day 97 Tuesday 2 November

Bunka in the morning and I watch the Melbourne Cup in the afternoon. I do some more work on the bike. No one can say I'm not doing enough exercise. Why don't my knees feel any better?

## Day 98 Wednesday 3 November

Six minutes on the bike and the knees feel surprisingly good. I then go for a walk around the tennis court and my left knee doesn't feel so bad. What's going on? I'm jubilant. Perhaps it's the severe talking to I gave it yesterday. I take Mum up to Innovations for her to buy a pair of white slacks and she buys me a nice outfit for Christmas. I must say buying clothes does cheer me up. I work on my computer in the afternoon. I still have rest times where I go and lie down with a book without feeling guilty. I remember Margaret's words of being kind to myself. I've managed to get through quite a bit of reading since the operation.

## Day 99 Thursday 4 November

As it is another cool day I decide to book another session in the rehab pool. Afterwards I go to the Mall to visit MBF to get a refund for the pool sessions I've had. I'm delighted to find I receive it all back. I work in the office and help Garnet in the afternoon.

## Day 100 Friday 5 November

Rain, rain and more rain! I know we need it but does it always have to rain on our tennis day? I spend ten minutes on the bike and my legs are very stiff. Later my left knee begins to hurt. It seems to catch me each time I walk. Then it goes away. I wonder what's causing that? Hopefully I'll get some answers on Monday.

## Day 101 Saturday 6 November

Same old Saturday. I really struggle up those steps at the building where I'm showing flats with my left knee paining. When I tell Mum later about my sore knee she suggests I take a Panadol and magically it seems to do the trick. I work on my photos all afternoon and do quite a number of pages. I want to show Justin and Karla my album when they come home at the end of the month. I enjoy creative memories and have achieved quite a lot in the time I've been doing it. It's amazing that I have enough photos to fill all those albums. Luckily Garnet was a prolific photographer when our children were young. They are wonderful memories and having to write a bit about each page makes it more informative. Hopefully the albums will be treasured by my children and will be something to show their offspring. Being able to use creative skills to make each page attractive is fun and I love it. I've decided to do one for Garnet's mother for her 100th birthday next year.

## Day 102 Sunday 7 November

Tomorrow is D-day when I find out whether I need to have my left knee done again or it's fine and dandy. Please let it be a good result. I don't want more surgery. I want to be able to enjoy Christmas without the threat of going back under the knife.

## Day 103 Monday 8 November

I walk tentatively into the doctor's surgery. I hope I don't have the long wait like last time but I'm prepared with a good book. There are a few before me so I settle in until I'm called. I didn't have to wait too long. The day of reckoning is here. What is to be my fate? Good news or bad? Up on the lighted screen are my X-rays and they both look identical. What is that big blob in the middle of each knee? Is that the prosthesis? Dr Walter walks in and greets me.

'Well Pam, I can't see any problems with either knee. The bone scan is fine as are your hips.' My heart starts to rejoice. 'Let me take a look.'

He moves both knees backwards and forwards and states that they are bending about the same. Good! I told him about the pain I had been getting in the right-hand corner of my left knee and he didn't really explain what that was. He told me my knees felt different because the problem in each knee was not the same and had to be tackled from different sides. My right leg had to be straightened as it was the one at a strange angle. Funny that it has turned out to be the better one. I must admit looking at the X-rays they both looked exactly the same.

His assistant came in while I was dressing and said that my knees would feel better at six months and better still at twelve. Perhaps I was rushing things. Maybe time is the greatest healer and what I am feeling is the surrounding tissue and nerve ends that have not yet settled down.

I leave the doctor's surgery feeling on top of the world. My knees are all right. Just get on with it Pam and ignore them. They will come good. I can't wait to tell Garnet the good news. I ring him and he rings Mum. She cried, he tells me later. I know she has been worrying about me and now she can relax as the news is good. My knees are fine! I drive straight to Warriewood Square to do my shopping and my knees feel great. Is it mind over matter? Maybe. I suppose on some days they'll be good and others not so good.

(I'm saying goodbye to my daily diary from here on. I will report each month until July next year on my progress.)

Chapter 7

# Life Goes On

## December 2004

The rest of November went by quickly with news of Justin and Karla's engagement just before they arrived on the 19th. Great jubilation! Garnet was involved in a drama with a tick bite that caused hospitalization. It was found that his heart was beating irregularly. He had to be placed on Warfarin much to his horror. No more drinking allowed. That was a blow especially as the festive season was approaching.

I attended my first meeting of the Society of Women Writers as publicity officer and was proud of the fact that I lasted through the two hours of the meeting, followed by the luncheon and guest speaker. It was so good being able to return to my normal activities. I played my first set of tennis during this month and I didn't play too badly for someone with stiff knees.

The welcome home party for Justin and Karla went well and it was a wonderful family day. We loved catching up on all the news. Also the early Christmas party was successful. I did a glazed ham for the first time and Garnet cooked it on his BBQ. It was delicious. We sat outside as it was a perfect day. Everyone relaxed and enjoyed the food and the company. Time went by quickly and soon Justin and Karla were on their way home again. I am always sad when Justin goes back to America.

I had the writing girls here for our Christmas get together and on the following Friday we had the tennis girls' Christmas luncheon. Everyone brought a plate and we had a varied array of goodies to choose from. I made a tuna dish that proved popular. I had to run off the recipe for the girls.

Sue Alexander and I did a little skit and I recited my poem.

## *NEW KNEES CLUB*

*I am the President of the New Knees Club,*
*To join this club, here is the rub,*
*Go into hospital and get new knees,*
*One or two, whatever you please*

*Five foundation members can unanimously say*
*They have a scar they can proudly display*
*Jan and Pam have one on each knee*
*In shorts obvious for all to see*

*Marg's the star we all admire*
*To see her run with her heart on fire*
*Chasing those balls around the court*
*That is what Bev and Norma also sought*

*I am the new kid on the block*
*Getting two done was quite a shock*
*So bend those knees, walk the miles*
*Put up with the discomfort and bloody well smile*

*You'll soon be ready to take your place*
*But will my knees stand the pace?*
*Of course they will, have no doubt*
*You might think differently when you hit the ball out*

*Has it been worth it, you may wonder*
*Or has it been a terrible blunder*
*Going under the knife*
*Not once but twice*

*Yes, it has as the weeks go by*
*And I can do more things when I really try*
*So watch me swing that racquet once more*
*Listen to the applause as I come out the door*

So fellow members we can celebrate today
We're back on the court without too much delay
To join our mates in the game we love
Let's drink to us all and the good Lord above.

The girls weren't in a hurry to leave and we sat around chatting after lunch. We had enjoyed our sets in the morning and it was wonderful being able to join in.

The next night was our Veterans Tennis Club's Christmas party. Garnet always goes into the fish markets to pick up the prawns and oysters. This year the oysters were HUGE. I always arrange beforehand what everyone will bring so we get a good choice in salads and sweets. Garnet cooked a piece of beef on his BBQ. There were 22 coming and as the night turned out to be cold we ate inside. For entertainment Ken played his flute while Lindsay sang some songs. I recited my poem. A fun night was had by all.

I am now at the five-month mark and I think I've done very well to get this far. I'm exercising every day, either walking or swimming or getting on the bike. I know I have to keep my knees flexible or they will stiffen up. I can walk long distances and I'm pleased about that. I'm trying to ignore my left knee. It doesn't feel like my right one but that's just the way it is. It may never feel any different but it's a hell of a lot better than it was.

I have a feeling 2005 is going to be a good year. No more dreaded operations to worry about. My tennis will improve as I get faster around the court. I will get on with my writing and other activities and help Garnet in his business. I feel optimistic about the future.

## January 2005

Here I am at six months with my knees still stiff and I am conscious of them all the time. They don't feel like my old knees and I don't think they ever will. I took myself off the anti-inflammatories for a week and my knees really stiffened up. My doctor put me on Mobic but they still felt the same so I discontinued those.

I was speaking to my friend Jan who is almost at 12 months since her operation and she is having the same problem. She went off her anti-inflammatories and her knees seized up like mine. She is back on them. We both came to the conclusion that our knees are never going to feel normal and we will just have to get used to them. At least we're not in pain and as I told her I have confidence they won't let me down when I'm running around the court. Yes, running! I can run and chase lobs again. That is such a good feeling. Although they feel stiff I just make them do what I want them to do and I don't suffer afterwards. I wish I could convince Jan to come back and play with us. She was such a good player but hasn't played in 11 years and doesn't want to begin now. She had been in a lot of pain before her operation and doesn't want to jeopardize her knees in any way. She does a lot of walking.

I keep thinking my knees will miraculously feel as they once did the more I exercise but there never seems to be a change. I get frustrated. You don't want them to seize up, Pam, so back on your bike!

## February 2005

I've gone back to my aqua aerobics at the Aquatic Centre at Frenchs Forest. I'm hoping this will help my knees become a little more flexible. We exercise in the deep water so we wear a floatie on our backs to keep upright in the water. We exercise for 45 minutes and we work hard, strengthening all parts of the body. The heart rate goes up and I sometimes find it hard to get my breath but it's getting easier the more I go. I'm attending two days a week but some of the ladies go every day. It's very popular. I feel fantastic when I come out.

I'm still getting on my bike as often as I can but my walking is curtailed at the moment as I hurt my right foot. I kicked it against a chair leg quite hard and it is still hurting two weeks after doing it. I had to come off the court on Friday as it hurt so much. It will get better and it doesn't hurt in the water.

## March 2005

I have been plugging away at my exercises and my knees don't feel any different. Still bloody stiff and my left one feels like a fence post most of the time. When I sit down for an extended period it takes a while to get moving again. I wish I knew what other people with new knees are experiencing. Maybe my knee is normal but then again maybe it's not. I have to go back in July to have it X-rayed and then a consultation with my specialist. I wish I could tell him how much I love my new knees but I don't think I'll be able to.

People ask how they are and I say just all right. I love aqua aerobics and enjoy doing all the exercises. Running in the deep water is good for my knees and it doesn't jar as on land. Walking is not so pleasurable although I do try to do it a couple of times a week. I get on the bike whenever I haven't done any of the above and I'm always glad when the ten minutes are up. No matter how much I do, the knees don't feel the slightest bit different. I suppose I think that magically one day they are going to feel normal but I think that day is a long way off. (I always seem to be complaining!)

## April 2005

It is nearly nine months since the operation. I'm plodding along and my knees feel about the same. I'm still doing the same exercise routine. I'm moving so much better on the court and now can move my feet into the correct position to hit the ball. I don't have to call 'yours' quite so often and I can get to short balls (well, perhaps not all). It's a great feeling and I realize how restricted I was before.

The one thing my left knee doesn't like is hard physical work around the garden. For the last two weekends I helped Garnet carry branches to the trailer and my knee complained afterwards. When I think back I can remember how my knees objected when we were cleaning up after the 1979 bushfire all those years ago. My knees have been a concern for quite a while. At least now I know they are strong enough to do the work whether they like it or not.

Chapter 8

# People with New Knees

## May 2005

At the end of April I decided to put a request in the "*Insearch*" column of the Daily Telegraph looking for people with new knees. I was interested in seeing how other people have coped. I was amazed at the response. Having so many great replies convinced me to go ahead and write my story. I asked for permission to include them. Most people were agreeable and even want a copy of the book.

I couldn't believe I would get such a response and it was so interesting reading their experiences, some good and some not so good. I couldn't wait to get to my computer each day to open my e-mail and see if there were any more to read. It made me feel better about myself. I didn't know there was a two percent chance of the operation failing but when you think about it, 98 percent success rate is pretty good! I suppose some have to be in the bottom two percent. Greg Pearce's letter that I mentioned in the preface is in that category. I emailed Greg months later just before the book was to be printed telling him his letter was included and asking how he was. This is his wife's reply.

*Dear Pam,*

*The replacement knees were not the trouble. It is because Greg's body makes too much calcium that forms straight away that is causing the problems. The last time he was in hospital in September last year, it was only a matter of hours so to speak that the knees seized up again. They took over a kidney bowl full of adhesions and bone out of both knees. He is only having the right one done this time and if it is not successful, he said that he would just have to bear it. I think it will be about fifth time he has been in all together. His doctor seems to think it will work, so here's hoping.*
*Bette Pearce.*

Oh boy, how unlucky can you be! Poor Greg, what he has had to go through. I do hope it is successful this time Greg. On the whole most of the people who e-mailed me had good stories to tell and were pleased with the outcome. Many are now playing their sports and most are pain free. That means a lot to so many people.
Here are some of their stories.

*Hi Pam,*
*My name is Carol McMaster. On 1 December 2004 I underwent bilateral unicompartmental knee joint replacement. I spent nine days in Fairfield Hospital (NSW). I went through physiotherapy. By the end of February 2005 my surgeon told me that my kneecaps were so badly worn that I would be left with permanent back pain and my mobility would always be severely restricted. As I was a nurse in my pre- operational life I had to retire on medical grounds as I am no longer able to lift, bend or attend to nursing duties.*

*It would be fair to say that my husband and I were looking forward to me having a 'normal life' however this was not to be. We were warned before the surgery that the success rate was 98%; I was unluckily in the other 2%. I bear my surgeon no malice as he did the best he could with the raw material he had to work with. I hope this is what you were looking for. If you need anything else please email me.*

*Regards,*
*Carol McMaster*
*Liverpool NSW*

I was sad to read this letter. It just goes to show how knees can be damaged in so many ways, at work or playing sport or just in usual wear and tear. I thank Carol for being honest as we need to hear both sides of the story. After replying to her she sent me another e-mail with more information and here it is.

*Hi Pam,*
*I am 50 years old. My knee problems were first diagnosed four years ago. At first I was told there was nothing that could be done because I wasn't old enough. As a nurse you are expected to lift heavy weights and do a lot of walking. I am only 5' 1 and a half and was expected to lift elderly patients many of whom were in excess of 18 stone. Over a period of time this resulted in wear and tear on my knees generally. As a result of the wear and tear the cartilage in my knees disintegrated my knees were rubbing bone on bone. I was also diagnosed with osteoarthritis as the knees weren't working properly, eventually it had an effect on my back. This has resulted in severe back pain.*

*Unicompartmental replacement is a replacement of the joints not the kneecaps. I am not bitter at my surgeon; he did everything possible for me. The operation was successful; it was the damage to the kneecap that could not be determined until I had the operation. My surgeon took a long time to warn me of the inherent risks; it just didn't work out. You can use my experience if you want to.*

*Regards,*
*Carol McMaster*

Good luck in the future Carol. I know how debilitating back pain can be. Think about massage as it helped me. I now have a back massage every fortnight to keep from having a problem.

*Dear Pam,*

*My name is Janifer and I'm 62 years of age. I had a total knee replacement four months ago and have no pain in the knee and am very pleased with how things are going. However, on walking a distance I find the leg gets tired and feels a bit heavy. I elected to have only one replaced at a time and also my doctor said he would only do it this way.*

*I found the first few days terrible and it took me about a week to be able to lift my leg off the bed. This was my main worry and I had very little bend in the knee. I was in hospital for one week and then Rehab for two weeks. I would recommend anyone contemplating this operation to go to a Rehab Hospital as they really make you work and get the muscles working again. I was the slowest out of my group at the beginning and was also one of the youngest but I caught up with them and was able to get around without a stick or assistance by the time I left Rehab.*

*I'm glad I did not do the two together as I have a terrace house with quite a few steps and apart from putting a railing on the curved steps I did not have to do anything else. By the time I arrived home I managed to do everything myself. I was really pleased to be able to get into the bath on the second night home as the hospital was telling me I'd have to have showers and needed a bath seat etc.*

*I feel that if I had done the two together I would have had to have assistance at home and would not have been able to get around so quickly. I had my first game of tennis at ten weeks and have since been playing once a week though not to the standard I was before as I'm still a bit nervous to jump or twist.*

*There was a woman in her early 80s in with me who had both knees together and she recovered amazingly well and had much better bends in her knees right from the beginning, compared to me. However, it took her a long time to be able to walk unaided.*

*I feel more information should be given to warn people how awful it is in the first few days and how much work is needed to get the knees bending. I was not expecting this. However, now I have done the one leg and know what to expect I'm not too worried about the other leg but am going overseas soon and hope the other holds out as long as possible as there is not too much pain and I feel like I need a holiday.*

*Hope you're progressing well.*

*Regards,*

*Janifer Zmak.*

Janifer has given good advice about going to a rehab hospital if you can. I found it invaluable. This is a good case for having one done at a time and most people have it done this way. Doctors prefer to do one and give you time to recover before having to do the second one but that means a longer period out of action. I'm pleased Janifer is not scared to go and have the other one done and I wish her well the second time around. Just glad it's not me!

*Dear Pam,*

*For some years I suffered extreme pain in my knees so much so that I could hardly walk and from a sitting position getting up was almost impossible. My husband Doug and I were raising a grandson (No 17th grandchild) who is 'Autistic Delay' and that upset me more because I couldn't do the things with and for him that I wanted to do. Finally, my doctor sent me to a specialist in Penrith. He examined me and said I needed both knees done, one knee full reconstruction and the other half knee. Then he said they would both have to be full reconstruction as the weight on my right knee would weaken with the extra work and carrying my weight as well as the tenderness from the operation on my left knee. I then asked if I could have them both done together. He was very hesitant as he said one other person had bilateral and he thought it would be too much for me but I was sure I could cope. Besides to come back for the second knee to be done would mean time away again and leaving the little fellow for my husband to look after alone would worry me.*

*The doctor agreed to do both knees together so I then went and booked into Nepean Hospital. I was put on a waiting list of 20 months. I received a letter from the hospital stating I was scheduled for the operation on 17 May 2003 but I had to have a full day with pre-op, testing and information regarding the procedure.*

*On 17 May I was operated on at 8.30am, then in the afternoon I walked to the toilet with a walking frame and I had physio at my bed daily. I continued to walk to the toilet, shower and around my bed. On the third day I was put on crutches and went out of the ward, up the hall and back. The following day I went to another room where they had a set of steps for walking up and down on crutches. The physiotherapist said, 'When you can walk up and down these steps you can go home.' I left hospital on the fifth day. I had the physio come to my home for ten days.*

*I had to go and see the specialist three weeks after the operation, then at six weeks. He said I was fine and to see him in a year and for me to attend the hospital three days a week for further physio. I did that for six weeks then I didn't have to go anymore. After my 12 month visit the doctor said I didn't need to come for another two years.*

*I have never felt better. I can run, jump, skip and above all I can dance with my dear little grandson to the Wiggles. He loves it. The only thing I cannot do is kneel down on my knees. It is certainly out of the question even on soft things. I really think they should tell you that before the operation just to prepare you for that everyday chore cannot happen anymore. I have healed beautifully. To look at my knees now the scarring is so faint and very fine you would never know it was done.*

*Believe me bilateral is definitely worth it!*

*Yvonne Williams*

I rang Yvonne after her letter arrived as she didn't have e-mail and this lady is one happy camper. She is 66 years old and admits she is a little overweight. She said that if you need something badly enough and you work at it from the beginning it will work for you. It certainly did for Yvonne. I can't believe she was out of bed the first day and home in five days. Her recovery was due to her hard work and the effort she put into rehab. Good on you, Yvonne. Now you can enjoy life with your fantastic grandson and husband Doug. Thanks for your inspirational letter.

*Hi Pam,*
*I noticed your request for information on double knee replacement recipients in last Saturday's Daily Telegraph. So, here I am, double knee replacements by Dr Merv Cross at the Mater Hospital seven years ago last January, back on the golf course within three months and have never looked back. Sure they are not your own in that they don't bend so far and there are certain restrictions like running etc., but I was in agony before the operation and my knees were governing my life.*
*I trust yours are working for you.*
*Paul Roberts.*

I felt good after reading this letter. Another sportsperson able to return to the game he loves. Paul was quite impressed when I told him I was back playing tennis and in his next e-mail he added a great story that I want to share with you.

*Dear Pam,*

*Back playing tennis doesn't sound too bad, that takes a fair amount of pressure and lateral movement. I had mine done at the age of 68, am now 75. Both of mine are pretty good, yes a little numbness at the knee cap and as I mentioned my maximum bend is around 125 degrees. I worked out at a pool every day for a couple of months, I found one at the Mowell Village at Castle Hill, which was reasonably cheap and devised my own exercises from the one visit to the Mater Physio at their pool.*

*When I had mine done the general consensus of opinion was that they would last ten years but my surgeon Merv Cross scoffed at that and reckons they will see me out and that no one really knows at this stage as the new techniques haven't been around for ten years. The only possibility that he did concede was that they may have to go in at some time or other to replace the plastic insert if it gets too worn.*

*Incidentally six months before my operation, Geoff Harvey the band leader from Channel Nine had his done, which was televised, angle grinders, saws, hammers, welding masks, the lot, again with Merv Cross at the Mater. Further to that after five years Merv called me in for an appraisal, reckoned that he had made a pretty good job and asked me whether I had any complaints, to which I replied, 'Only one, it hasn't improved my golf.'*

*He looked at me for a while and then said, 'You have given me an idea. If I organised a golf day for all my knee recipients, would you be in it?' 'Of course,' I replied.*

*So two years ago about 50 of us assembled at The Australian Golf Club for lunch, golf, drinks and dinner for both recipients and their partners all on Merv. Now that's a good news story for your book. It could only happen in Australia where ex-footballers, business-men and women, people from all walks of life and of course Geoff Harvey, all gathered around the grand piano singing away, at the invitation and I might add expense, of a world renowned orthopaedic surgeon. Trust I have been of some help,*
*Regards,*
*Paul Roberts.*

Isn't that a simply marvellous story! Good on you Dr Merv Cross! Can you imagine if you hadn't operated on those 50 guys they would now be at home bothering their wives, moaning and groaning, instead of out on the golf course. I don't know whether I would like to have seen Geoff Harvey's operation. A little too much blood and gore for my liking. What's this about angle grinders, saws and hammers? Surely they weren't used on me? Were they?

I contacted Geoff for permission to use his name in the above story and asked him if he would like to contribute his experiences for my book. He told me his wife Katrina would be better at writing it and as she stayed at the hospital each day with Geoff she would have witnessed first-hand what he went through and what sort of patient he was. As most men are wimps as far as pain is concerned, she was there to make sure he did as he was told. It must have been a scream nursing Geoff and lucky for other patients as his sense of humour carried the day and saw him through the worst of it. Thank you Geoff and Katrina for sharing your story with me and now the reader.

*Hi Pam,*

*Geoff has asked me to send off a few words to you regarding his knee replacements back in 1997. Firstly, he is more than happy for you to include the story of him playing the piano at the big 'knee golf day'. It was quite an amazing thing to do but Merv Cross really is quite an amazing man. Geoff, as you are probably aware, had two knee replacements done at once. I must confess that this was more at my urging than Geoff's inclination because I figured I would have a much greater battle getting him to return for the second operation. As it turned out, it was the most sensible for Geoff. It wasn't a case of twice the pain but rather half the length of time.*

*In fact, to be honest, Geoff doesn't even recall very much pain at all - thank god for those drugs. As it was the first time he had ever been to hospital he was, needless to say, extremely apprehensive but turned out to be a model patient.*

*I virtually moved into the hospital with him also so was able to follow it all very closely and help him with the physio when the nurses (who were wonderful) were too busy. I also was able to keep a good timing on his drugs and make sure he had his dosages right on time, before the pain kicked in.*

*His sense of humour was extraordinary the whole way through and his determination to get up and out of there was extraordinary. I think it was the day after the operation, when he had literally just been sent to his room after the ICU, that he insisted on having a shower. The nurses were not particularly enthusiastic about this but he was adamant and just wanted to start feeling back to normal again. With my help and another strong nurse, and a good drenching for all of us, he did achieve this albeit looking very pale at the time. The hardest part of the whole healing process for Geoff, was the physiotherapy. However, Merv had instructed from the outset that unless he was prepared to do it properly, Merv was not going to perform the operation. In Geoff's case, unlike most Australian men, he had never set foot in a gym before let alone 'worked out'. He had played a bit of Rugby but never very seriously. (He won't like me saying that.) Anyway, the long and short of this was that he found it pretty tough going and when some of the muscles (which hadn't been used for quite a while) started to hurt, he was convinced there was a major problem and that the operation had been a failure. We had to explain the 'no pain, no gain' theory to him. He actually really enjoyed the hydrotherapy and was diligent with this. We came straight down to Berrima when he was discharged, even though we had a townhouse in Sydney (three storeys high! Not appropriate.) and fortunately, the Bowral Private Hospital had a great physio centre and hydrotherapy pool so we were able to go there every day for the duration and it was no real effort.*

*One of the funny things I remember when Geoff was at the Mater was when he was doing his routine walks around the ward, getting everything mobilized, he would have a chat to all and sundry and ask them what they were in for. If it was knees, he would have no hesitation in calling them 'gutless' or words to that effect, if they were only having one done instead of two. He did bring a lot of humour to the ward and the nurses would occasionally ask him to wander around to someone's room to give them a bit of a cheer-up and buck-up.*

*Of course, it was also a bit 'circus' like in that '60 Minutes' taped Geoff's whole procedure, including the operation, before and after. Geoff is very proud of the fact that it was a huge ratings winner for Channel Nine when it went to air and I must say he did give them a good performance.*

*Pam, if there is anything else I can help you with, don't hesitate to e-mail me and good luck with the book. We've had many, many people ringing over the years, and wanting to talk to Geoff, and even me, about the whole operation, so I think you have a ready market.*
*Kind regards,*
*Katrina Harvey*

I can just imagine Geoff telling everyone who had only one knee or one hip replacement 'gutless'. People who have a bilateral do think we're a cut above the rest and so heroic for going the whole hog. Katrina certainly played a big part in Geoff's decision to have it done in the first place and his inspiration in the rehabilitation period. Katrina, you deserve a medal. You too, Geoff!

*Hi Pam,*

*Grahame had both his knees replaced about three years ago. He had the operation done at Gosford in the Brisbane Waters Private Hospital, Woy Woy NSW. He coped very well with the operation and the usual medication, but after a few days refused pain medication (never taken a Panadol in his life - not even for a hangover). After his main stay in hospital he attended physio at Woy Woy General Hospital where he was given an exercise routine. He also attended the Hydro heated pool at the same place.*

*After being discharged from hospital he continued with exercise. He was lucky enough to have a mate who was a physio and owned his own practice and he gave him advice on what exercises to do. If he said to do 20, Grahame did 40. He also attended the local public heated pool everyday where he did lots of knee bends and walking up and down the pool. Grahame coped very well with the whole thing. He was back driving the car within three weeks. He is pain free, swims a lot and looks after the pool, does heaps and heaps of gardening.*

*Hope this helps, if you need anything else please let me know.*

*Regards,*
*Jean Kennedy*

Thank you Jean for telling me about your husband. He sounds a very determined man wanting to get back his mobility as soon as possible. With the right attitude it is possible to be up and running in no time (well, almost no time). I wish him all the best and how lucky for you he can still do all the gardening.

*Hi Pam,*
*I had both knees replaced at the Mater Hospital in February 2003 by Dr Merv Cross. My father-in-law also had both of his replaced seven years ago. What do you want to know?*

*Regards,*
*Robert Woods*
*Griffith*

I replied to Robert and asked for more detail which he generously gave in his next e-mail.

*Hi Pam,*
*I had bowed legs which meant that my weight (and there is a fair bit of it) wasn't supported by my legs and the knees took the majority of it on the edges and subsequently wore them out. I had bone on bone at 58. I was flat out walking to the local shops - about 300 metres - without difficulty and a lot of pain.*

*When Dr Cross operated, he also straightened out the legs, much to my surprise. Apparently, it is in the way they cut the bone and insert the joint. It is much better now. I didn't go to rehab, as I reckoned that if my father-in-law could do exercises at home (he was 76) I could do it also.*

*I had a lot of visits to the physio as I also developed a blood clot, a varicose vein blew up, and a lot of visits to the local pool, walking in the water. The rest I did myself at home. I was walking without the aid of crutches or sticks in five weeks.*

*As I live in Griffith, my wife and sister drove me home direct from hospital, the trip took about ten hours (with stops, and there were a lot of them) I wanted to get home as I was missing the grandkids badly and we also had tickets to John Farnham's last show. (I never got there but my mother-in-law enjoyed my ticket.) My knees still get stiff, particularly if I sit too long. The left knee is not as good as the right one, but they are better than what I had before. I walk most mornings about five to six km and experience no problems.*

*What I miss most is not being able to kneel. I find that I am lying on the floor to do things down low. You should have seen me trying to paint the skirting boards, marvellous what you can do with a long handled paintbrush. My knees still have pins and needles and not much feeling on the outside. They tell me that it can take up to three years for all the nerves to grow back. I am now 61 years old. No, my father-in- law will not have to have his done again as he is now 82.*

*I think the hardest part was the first couple of days after the operation. The brain is a powerful thing, isn't it? It tells you that it is going to hurt like hell when you go to stand, and for a couple of days I physically couldn't get out of the chair without help. My sister has a bad knee also but at this time is refusing to get it fixed as she reckons that she could not do the physio like I did. You have to do the work or the whole exercise has been a waste of time.*

*In closing, I am certainly glad that I have bitten the bullet and had the operation as my quality of life has improved dramatically.*

*Regards,*

*Robert Woods*

A lot of what Robert told me is similar to my experience. The fact that one knee is not as good as the other. Sorry you missed John Farnham's concert but I'm glad the ticket wasn't wasted. Kneeling is a problem and when I do gardening, I sit on my bottom but I must look a sight when getting up. I resemble a giraffe with stiff legs. Hence, I don't do much gardening.

*Hi Pam,*

*I couldn't help noting your request for contact from others who have had new knees. I had my right knee replaced on 4 May 2004 and eventually returned to work in the first week of September 2004 (total of 16 weeks off). I had to have the operation as I was in constant pain from the knee joint which just kept getting worse. I'd also developed a 'bandy-legged' look. The leg was straightened when the knee was replaced - and although I am now not in any significant pain, I am unable to bend the knee past 80-85 degrees. Following the initial surgery, my knee remained very swollen for a long time and I think this created a situation where scar tissue and other deposits prevented satisfactory movement. In July 2004 my knee was 'manipulated' under anaesthetic in an effort to produce more 'bend'. There was improvement in bending immediately after this procedure - but as soon as the swelling returned so too did the lack of bend and the degree of bend remained at 80-85 in spite of fairly intense physio and hydrotherapy.*

*In December, my specialist did an arthroscopy in order to remove scar tissue etc. and tried again to help 'free up' the new knee. Once more, swelling after this procedure limited the immediate post procedure movement and when it eventually subsided, I was back to around 85 degree movement. I'm glad I had the knee done as I now only have problems climbing stairs when the lack of knee bend is a 'hassle'. My left knee is not yet as bad as my right one was - and I'm certainly not in any hurry to go through it all again. I have learnt from my experience that everyone responds differently regardless of whether you're fat, skinny, middle-aged or elderly. By the way, I'm now 59 years of age and hope my good knee can last well into my 60s.*

*I hope my information is of some value to you in writing your story - and I sincerely hope your double knee replacement is proving to be successful for you.*

*Regards,*
*Rae Bylsma*

Rae, I certainly hope your good knee gives you a few more years before having to go through it all again. It is amazing the number of people that have to have the knee manipulated under anaesthetic to give it more bend. I wonder why? I'm glad that didn't happen to me.

*Dear Pam,*
*I was born 1/9/52 and had a hereditary arthritic condition called Spondylo Epiphiseal Dysplasysia Tarda (not sure of spelling) which affects all my joints. As a young teenager I showed stiffness and did not have the flexibility of others my age. At age 13 I had the first of many operations on my joints. My right elbow had to have pieces of bone removed that had come away from the joint.*

*At age 33 in 1986 and two young children (three & five), I had my right hip replaced and then three months later had my left hip replaced by Dr Bill Walter. This became very necessary since my quality of life had become so compromised and I was in considerable pain. Relief was immediate but I was on crutches for six weeks after both operations and in those days the joint was not allowed to take any weight for that time.*

*In 1991 my right hip replacement wore out and I was forced to have a hip revision where they put a new socket in (eight weeks on crutches and no weight on the joint). It was found that the type of replacement that was originally put in was not as successful as the type that had been put in my left hip three months later in 1986.*

*In 1999 my left hip replacement wore out and Bill Walter carried out a total hip revision of it. In regards to these revisions I believe it has been stated that young people are more active and in a sense harder on their new joints than a sedentary 75 year old and hence have to be prepared to get their joints redone.*

*In 2002 (aged 50) I had bilateral knee replacements. I reached a stage in my life again where I was in so much pain and could not stand for any length of time and my left knee kept giving way that something had to be done. I convinced Dr Bill Walter that I wanted to have both knees done together to cut down on recovery time. This was the best decision ever and I would recommend it to anyone who is in reasonable health. My life totally changed and I feel now I can do almost anything. At the moment walking is such a pleasure, whereas beforehand my time was spent calculating how to cut down walking anywhere. My physical condition has improved dramatically.*

*Before the operation I made sure I had good muscle condition. I had been doing aqua aerobics since 1987 but increased the number of classes per week to help my fitness. Deep water aqua is a fabulous non jarring exercise and I would recommend it to anyone with bad joints. The right knee behaved beautifully and was fitted with a non cemented prosthesis; however, the left would not stop moving around and was consequently cemented. The recovery after the operation was good. Continual movement of the operated joint is essential otherwise it apparently will seize up. Hence, they put you on a dreaded machine to keep your knee continually moving. This I found quite difficult and even complaining I was uncomfortable brought no response and next morning when they finally stopped it they found the cut had opened so I had to go back to theatre to have it restitched! I had 11 days in hospital and then rather than go to rehab I was able to come straight home. I returned to the hospital two days later to have a session of physio in the pool where they taught me all the exercises that I needed to do. I forced myself in all weathers to get in our freezing pool and do them daily and also go for a short walk up the street. I found that by my six week checkups I was going really well and able to swap my crutches for a stick.*

*I believe that one should hold off having joint replacement operations until you can't take it any longer. It seems they only have a limited life and being only in my 50s I know that I will have to have them done again. On saying that, my quality of life so improved that I believe it is totally worth it.*

*Regards,*
*Pam Thompson*

I met Pam at the Warringah Aquatic Centre when I began going to help my fitness before my knee operation. She was so positive and helpful to me as I was preparing to have it done. Not once did she put the negative side but told me how good I'll be afterwards. I didn't go back to aqua aerobics until I was at the six month mark and all the girls were pleased to see me with my brand new straight legs. It's hard to hide a crooked one in a bathing suit. I remember being so happy walking in that first day. I asked Pam if she would write something about her operation for my book and she kindly consented. She presents a very good case of getting two done at once. She has been through a lot and I admire her tenacity and bravery facing up to all those operations but to see her in the pool with a big smile I know she will not be too concerned at having to go through it again. Thanks Pam for your contribution.

*Dear Pam,*

*My operation was performed by Dr Mervyn Cross (no relative) at the Mater Hospital in June 2001. As anticipated, there was a fair amount of pain which was made bearable by various pain killers. After a week in hospital during which time I received some early physiotherapy I was then transferred to Hunters Hill Rehab Hospital for ten days. The physiotherapy here was more intense causing a higher level of pain but as there were several others who had had similar operations, hips, knees etc. we managed to make light of it, coupled with a sense of humour. I asked one of the physios how long the pain would last and she told me 'six weeks'. I found this to be 'spot on'. Living in a block of units I found the flat concrete floor of the garage space to be a good place to practise my walking with the aid of crutches. After two weeks I ventured outside with a walking stick and increased day by day the distance walked until I was able to walk without my stick. I then considered my rehabilitation complete. I do not find my knees unduly stiff but realising they are not as efficient as natural knees they are an excellent alternative. I am now 83 and find that I have a hip degeneration requiring replacement. I will discuss with the orthopaedic surgeon the possibility of an operation as soon as possible and can only hope that this will be as successful as the knees.*

*I hope this information will be of some help towards your book that you are writing and wish you every success.*

*Yours sincerely,*

*Colin Cross*

It was lovely receiving Colin's letter as he didn't have e-mail. Many of the things he mentioned I could relate to and considering his age I think he is going very well. I wish you well Colin with your hip operation but I think you'll find it a breeze after knees. I rang and spoke to him as he gave me his phone number. I admired his attitude and how much he is enjoying being able to do things he couldn't do before. Good for you, Colin!

*Dear Pam,*

*Playing tennis must be a miracle! I don't have much balance and couldn't run if I tried... The Revision as they call it is a much more serious op than just the replacement. A Revision is to replace the cement and bone that is crumbling (helped by falling off a ladder) and in my case to put a longer pin in my thigh. I am only just over 5'1" and a bit on the heavy side - certainly not svelte. I think weight isn't a good go. I sleep with a soft slim pillow between my knees as I can't bear the weight of one knee on the other... These knees weigh a ton... Once asleep the pillow ends up on the floor or the other side of the bed... I had nothing but the best of treatment both in the hospital and the Rehab. It was a bit like Hollywood but with the highest standard of care physios could impart.*

*I really gave it my all (don't overdo things I was told) but my knees were in such bad shape before the Op and I had lost a lot of muscle quality or simply just lost the muscle completely like one of my quads and now the calf muscles aren't what they should be.*

*I was only given the facts that a bilateral was what was needed and I do agree with that. The revision was a different kettle of fish they would only do one at a time even though I requested to have both done simultaneously.*

*I am retired and live in Hay in NSW on a sheep station where I just potter with dogs, chooks and some gardening...*

*Over to you now and I don't mind what you write in your book.*
*Regards,*
*Claire McFarlane*

After reading this letter I realized how fortunate I am being able to run around a tennis court. What Claire would give to be able to do that or something equally as physical. We wish Claire a happy life with her dogs and chooks on her sheep station in Hay.

*Hello Pam,*
*I read your article in the Daily Telegraph about knees. I had both my knees replaced two and a half years ago and they have been terrific. I do work for a specialist so knew that the operation would only be a success if I did a lot of preparing and after work. I think a lot of patients think that the surgeon is a miracle worker and by replacing the knees they will be fine. Not so. I worked with a physio for nine months before my operation, trying to get all my muscles, tendons etc. as supple as possible so they would spring back into place as quickly as possible after the trauma of surgery. It took a lot of work, physio once a week, gym three times a week and swimming three times a week. I couldn't walk much at this stage so all these things were necessary.*

*After the op which I didn't find too traumatic, probably the first three days after surgery, then I was able to hop our of bed, walk a few paces with a frame and by day five, I could swing my own legs out of bed with a bandage so felt quite free. By week three, I was back to the physio for more work on my knees, breaking up all the scar tissue and loosening all the muscles. I also started hydro therapy three times a week.*

*By week five, no crutches, still visiting the physio each week and a masseur the off week, I was also back swimming twice a week at this stage. I started back playing golf after four months and haven't looked back. I still swim three times a week and play golf twice a week. I am now 58 years old and will probably have to have them done again when I'm about 70. My condition was past the point of no return, osteo-arthritis, no cartilages left, they had disintegrated, and spurs growing into each other, also the patella had worn out. I can only put it down to too much sport as a youngster. I would recommend it to anyone with severe knee problems. My husband's reaction was that it was great not to see the pained expression on my face anymore. I hope this helps you with your research.*
*Val Avent*
*ACT*

This letter gives so much good advice to prospective patients thinking of having a knee replaced. The work you do beforehand is equally as important as the work you do afterwards. My friend Jan told me to build up my quadriceps so I did a lot of leg lifts before I had my operation and it certainly helped. It's good to hear Val is enjoying her sports again and her husband is enjoying seeing her out of pain. Good on you Val!

*Dear Pam,*

*My sister-in-law forwarded me your request for info on people who had both knees replaced together. I fall into that category, having had the operation on the 8 Nov 04. My problems started while I was in the Air Force, having both medial cartilages removed in 1960 and 1961. I was problem free up until 15 years ago when the pain gradually increased over time, until I could no longer bear it. I was also very restricted in what I could do.*

*I saw the specialist with X-rays who decided after discussion, that the only way to go was with both knees replaced together. The operation was without complications; the only drama on the first night was blood loss from the drains in both knees, necessitating blood transfusions. I had already donated blood for the op, which was administered during the procedure.*

*The epidural was removed on the third morning, leaving me with considerable pain which was dampened with a shot of Morphine and again on the fourth morning. All other pain control was by capsule, affectionately called Aussie Pills, because of the green and yellow colouring. Don't remember the correct name. The op was on the Monday afternoon; my first walk in the 'frame' was on Wednesday afternoon, which was an anti-climax due to absence of any real pain or trauma. My crutches arrived the same afternoon and first walk with them was on the Thursday morning with the physio directing. I found it easier to use them in the walking mode, rather than both together! I found them and the walking to be no problem. The hardest was getting out of bed and into bed for the first few days. Once I mastered that without risk of falling, I spent more time out of bed than in, as I had sore buttocks, heels and elbows.*

*I was released to come home on the Tuesday, the eighth day, with visits planned to the physio in a couple of days. Also they planned some hydrotherapy, with a list of exercises I continued in our own pool. About two weeks after the op, I stretched my left leg to lock it, when the hamstring let go with a shot of pain that had me out of bed cursing. About three days later, my wife said, 'What is the dark mark on the back of your leg?' There was a near black mark from the groin to the back of the knee, about 100mm wide where it had bled. The soreness only lasted a few days, which I was pleased about. I also had suture abscesses form on the right wound, which went away in a week after antibiotics.*

*I still have some numbness on the outside of both knees, which the specialist said will eventually go away. I find myself doing lots of things I found difficult before, without effort, though I get niggles occasion-ally when squatting and on steep ground and steps. Just a reminder of the trauma that has happened.*

*Hope this helps with your research, and if you have further questions, please feel free to ask.*

*Regards,*
*Bernie Forrest*

I too had to have three blood transfusions after the operation as I had lost a lot of blood. I hadn't donated any of my own as some people do but was perfectly happy with what I was given. I also have the numbness on the outside of both knees. I'm glad Bernie is now able to do lots of things he couldn't do before. It obviously was well worth going through the pain to get the good result. Good luck, Bernie!

*Dear Pam,*

*Over seven months ago, I had double knee replacements. On the week of my operation Channel 7 was preparing a programme on knee replacements and I was asked via my surgeon if I was willing to be interviewed and my operation videoed. This took place but it was about three months before it was shown on Today Tonight and of course only short excerpts from all that was filmed. I was so positive about the whole experience because I was in a lot of pain walking, standing and barely able to climb the stairs at home at the end of the day. I had completely worn my knees out, never sparing myself over the years; climbing, walking etc. on our many holidays here and overseas.*

*When I think how positive I was in that interview I am glad they are not asking me now how I feel! I expected that by diligently doing my exercises at home and at the pool, I would gradually be walking normally and painlessly again. Now seven months later that is far from reality. My knees are still so tight that walking is difficult and puts great strain on my back and leg muscles. There has been no recognisable improvement over the last few months and I feel trapped in this condition and wonder if I will ever be able to lead the life I was able even before the operation. I am told it could take up to 12 months but I would welcome the encouragement of any improvement at the moment.*

*I am 62 and enjoy working three days a week in a stimulating environment which I returned to after eight weeks of 'sick leave'. Although my work does not suffer, having been in the same position for 14 years, some days I am so exhausted and sore I wonder if I should leave but wonder how I would fill my time meaningfully when there are few things I am able to enjoy with such poor mobility. So to date the whole experience has been very disappointing but I really had no choice. I don't think one knee at a time was ever a good option for me and doubt it would have made a difference in the long run. Currently I exercise daily, go to the physio twice a week and he encourages me on two pieces of gym equipment. I am also resuming aqua aerobics which I have enjoyed in the past.*

*I felt depressed the first few weeks after the operation but got over that as I found things to do that interested me: patchwork, quilting and cross-stitch which I had not had much time for over recent years. I was hopeful for a gradual improvement but as time has passed and I get around and try to do as much as I can, I recognize nothing much has changed and it is hard to know when it will. I am very fortunate in having a wonderful husband to help me but do not take advantage of that and pull my weight in doing as much as I can. A daughter helps with housework and gardening fortnightly. I can drive, stand more patiently and climb the stairs but walking for any length of time will guarantee that the next day I am stiff and sore.*

*On my last visit to the surgeon, he said everything was progressing normally and he wouldn't need to see me until December. I don't know anyone who has had such a long recuperation but maybe it is normal. I certainly wasn't prepared in any way for such a long recovery. I guess I have been stopped in my tracks after a very active life despite increasingly painful walking which I just ignored as much as possible. I suppose it is a great learning curve and as I am often reminded there are people far worse off than I am!*
*Name withheld at writer's request (name supplied)*

I can sympathise with this person as I too didn't think I was ever going to be normal again. With all the exercise I was doing I thought that miraculously they would come good but that was not the case. Let's hope this person gets back to her active pursuits soon. I'm sure she's pleased she had them both done together and doesn't have to face another long period of rehabilitation.

*Dear Pam,*

*My name is Shirley Hawkins, I'm 76 and I live at Leonay. I had my knees replaced in April 2003 and am thrilled with the result. I had been unable to walk further than about 50 yards without sitting down and couldn't stand up to do anything for more than a few minutes and had been on a walking stick for about six or seven years. Now I am able to go shopping again (my wonderful husband used to do all that) and can stand for ages. I still have times when my legs feel stiff, especially in the morning when I get out of bed and I also have found that one leg is better than the other, but I don't think I will ever play tennis again like you can. I am loathe to kneel down but I think it is mostly that I'm scared to and I had a scary experience when I tried to retrieve something that had rolled under the bed. I sat on the floor and couldn't get back up again, and as my husband was away until the next evening, and it was 11 o'clock at night I thought I was stuck there for the night. I wriggled my way from the bedroom to the stairs and was able to sit on the top step and let my legs down a couple of steps and found that there's always a way to get out of trouble. I guess you have had plenty of these types of experiences. Nice to communicate with you.*
*Regards,*
*Shirley Hawkins*

I loved the part about trying to stand from a sitting position and finding you couldn't. I can relate to that. It's a frightening prospect. I try not to sit on the floor as it is difficult standing up as you can't turn around and put any weight on the front of your knees. I am happy that Shirley has found her mobility again and can enjoy shopping and other activities. Like you I still have the stiffness but the more I use them it wears off during the day.

*Dear Pam,*

*I spotted the note in the 'Tele' last month re your quest for first-hand reports on the outcomes of knee surgery, and I'm happy to contribute.*

*Mine took place just seven years ago (05-05-98) in Berkeley Vale Private - and it couldn't have been better. The hospital and its staff were wonderful, my doctor did a brilliant job and the outcome has been totally satisfactory.*

*Having said that, I trust I can make a useful contribution for the benefit of future patients - my doctor and I did not see eye-to-eye on the benefits of the postop physio. While he - and the nurses - were adamant that I would not be discharged until I had achieved a 90degree bend, I was equally adamant that such an aim was impossible and I refused to go beyond the preliminary stages of the physio torture programme, despite the threat of being kept there until I conformed I didn't mind staying on - I liked the place, liked the people, liked the food - in fact, couldn't wait to get there again - which I did in 2001 for a prostatectomy.*

*I pointed out to the doctor and the nurses that I may not know as much as they do about surgery, but I do know a little about engineering, and you can't compress a fluid, which, with my knee inflated to football size, is precisely what they were trying to do.*

*So, having left hospital at the appointed time, I concentrated on getting my knee straight while I walked (a tip I'd been given by another, second-time, patient), and let the bending follow. Which it did over about a two month period with the minimum of pain and angst and the maximum of bend - 110 degrees, thank you very much.*

*On each of the occasions I went back for an annual check-up my doctor expressed his pleasure and satisfaction at the condition of the knee, which continues to serve me well, with no adverse after-effects. Following this, I tell my story to every prospective patient I happen to meet - and there are many, as you know - and to date haven't had anybody come back to tell me it didn't work.*

*So that's my story - I hope it's of interest and value.*

*Kind Regards,*

*C. Max Stahl*

*Arcadia Vale NSW*

Thanks Max, you have given some good advice. I can imagine how difficult it would be trying to get your knee, the size of a football to bend and how painful. I didn't have the swelling so the bending wasn't quite as torturous as yours must have been. I'm pleased you were able to get it to bend eventually with perseverance and exercise.

*Dear Pam,*

*Thank you for your e-mail, I will now attempt to answer your questions in detail as follows:*

a. *Cost - yes it cost me personally about $4,000.00 but I did claim excess medical expenses that year which further reduced my actual cost by another $500.00 or so.*

b. *Use of Costing - yes that would be fine, provided names were not used, and medical staff could not guess who was being used in the example.*

c. *Sharing Experiences - yes I would be happy to share experiences, for example at my first review I mentioned that my toes on both feet were progressively becoming numb - Merv Cross advised that this had nothing to do with the new knees! I have often wondered if others experienced the same symptoms.*

d. *Rehab & Currently - before my operation, Merv Cross suggested I get fit and lose about ten kg from my then 103 kg body - I am 180 cm (just over six ft.) tall. This I did with dieting and swimming about 3/4 km each day for three months. For my Rehab I took to the water again after about three weeks and haven't looked back since. I am exercising quite regularly and keeping the weight around 95 kg. I believe I am probably quite fit relative to other 60 yr old Australian males.*

e. *In Retrospect - yes I am pleased with the result and quite glad that I had the operation. Before the op I could not stand at a desk, or walk around shopping centres etc. for more than an hour or so without aching knees/legs. Now, I can do these things for eight hours without concern. I can kneel down and I have more angular movement than before the op.*

f. *Golfing - no, I am not a keen golfer, but I do remember Merv Cross mentioning something about golf at my first (12 month) review. I believe I have another automatic review at the five years mark. Maybe I will then be invited to golf?*

g. *Age - I have just turned 60 yrs (2 March) and I was57 yrs at the time of operation. I sold my business and retired about six months before the op. I could not have contemplated the op whilst running my own business.*

h. *Knee Longevity - this has been my one fear all along. Clearly at 57 yrs I was one of the younger clients for Merv Cross and he suggested that the new knees would last about 15 yrs. This would put me around 72 yrs and not really looking forward to another op. Merv also suggested that by then the refurbishing procedure would be well developed and relatively minor. I can only hope he is correct!*

i. *Sporting Activity - no, I am not involved in any organised sport, but I do have a small gym for walking, cycling etc. permanently set up downstairs. I use this four to five days each week. We also have a heated pool which is suitable for lap swimming, and we have a beach (Forster) about 500 m from our front door which we use for long walks. There is also an indoor heated pool locally which I plan to use again during the winter months (if winter ever comes this year!).*

*If I can be of further assistance, please ask and I would be happy to oblige.*

*Has anyone else commented on numb toes after the operation?*
*Regards,*
*Trevor Fardell*

Thanks for your comprehensive reply, Trevor. You have covered so many questions people often ask but I'm not sure about the numb toes. I have a tingly feeling in my right ankle that I put down to the operation. I'm sure it will go away in time.
I had it when I had my varicose veins done a number of years ago. I cursed my doctor at the time. Trevor also sent me a costing of his operation and he kindly has allowed me to include it for your information. Over and above all other costs Trevor was out of pocket about $4000 after his health fund and Medicare had given their refunds.

He also got some back through his taxes. Mine cost me close to $7000. I'm hoping to get some back through my tax at the end of the financial year. (I did receive over $2,400 in my tax return leaving me out of pocket about $4,600). Thanks again Trevor and may you have many more years before anything has to be done. Let's not think about that!

I hope the above letters have been of some help to you as they were to me. I can't thank those kind folks enough for going to the trouble of e-mailing me and also giving me permission to share their experiences with the reader.

## BILATERAL TOTAL KNEE REPLACEMENT - COSTS SUMMARY

| Date | Amount | Description | Medicare Refund | Health Fund Refund | Residual Cost to TJF |
|---|---|---|---|---|---|
| 4-Dec-02 | $155.00 | Surgeon's Consult. Fee | $58.95 | N/A | $96.05 |
| 16-Jan-03 | $230.00 | Physician's Pre Op. Medical exam | $125.55 | N/A | $104.45 |
| 3-Feb-03 | $5,275.00 | Surgeon's Operating Fee | $1,407.90 | $469.25<br>*(Into Bev's Bank A/c)* | $3,397.85 |
| 3-Feb-03 | $356.20 | Surgeon's Assistant | $281.60 | | |
| 14-Feb-03 | $850.00 | Anaesthetic services | $298.35 | $99.45 | $452.20 |
| 16-Jan-03 | $506.00 | Physiotherapists Fee | N/A | $307.00 | $199.00 |
| 6-Feb-03 | $452.70 | Pathology | $197.75 | $65.70 | Nil - No Gap |
| 11-Feb-03 | $404.30 | In Hosp. X - Rays (New Knees)<br>PLUS<br>Doppler No 1 (X-Ray for clotting) | $243.95 | $57.95<br>*(Into Bev's bank A/c)* | $102.40 |
| 12-Feb-03 | $85.00 | Physician's In Hosp Visit (Clotting) | $45.95 | $15.30 | $23.75 |
| 2-Feb-03 | $544.50 | Accommodation | N/A | $480.00 | $64.50 |
| 28-Feb-03 | $78.95 | Hire of Chair & walking Aids | N/A | $78.95 | Nil |
| 11-Feb-03 | $23,888.95 | Mater Hospital Fee<br>*(Priv. Hlth Fund "Top Cover")* | N/A | 23588.95 | $300.00<br>*(Hlth Fund Surcharge)* |
| 19-Feb-03 | $182.00 | Doppler No 2 (X-Ray for clotting) | $132.00 | N/A | $50.00 |
| TOTAL | $33,008.60 | | $2,792.00 | $25,162.55 | $4,790.20 |

Chapter 9

# How the Prosthesis is Made

## June 2005

After receiving Paul Roberts' e-mail about the golf day with Dr Merv Cross and his patients I wrote to Dr Cross asking permission to use the letter in my book. He agreed and then gave me the name of Dr Greg Roger, the manufacturer of the prosthesis he uses in his knee operations. I rang to make an appointment to see him. Dr Roger is the Managing Director of ASDM (Australian Surgical Design and Manufacture) at St Leonards. I took Margaret with me as I knew she would be interested to see what is actually in our knees and what goes into the making of them. Dr Roger made us very welcome and invited us into his office for a talk before taking us around the factory.

Dr Roger is an engineer as well as a doctor and assists Dr Cross every Monday with knee replacements to keep his hand in and stay close to patients' requirements. In 1992 he began designing and making the prosthesis that is used today. He is also making and designing other allied components. He showed us his design which we could feel and see how heavy it was and how shiny. It weighs about 430g and the other piece that goes underneath weighs 150g. Wow, no wonder my knees felt heavy in the first instance! He did explain that the amount of bone that is cut away to fit the prosthesis weighs around about the same so that made me feel a bit better.

Dr Roger explained how knees were done in the 60s, 70s and 80s and were not as good as hips but in the 90s the procedure was perfected and the results were much better. It was Dr John Charmley who did the first hip operation back in the late 50s in England. We have certainly progressed a long way since then. Many of the early ones were done with cement which crumbled and had to be done again. Dr Cross uses screws to secure the polyethylene (white plastic that sits on the titanium) to the tibia. Some doctors use screws and some don't. Some still use cement. Dr Walter uses a stem instead of screws. The top section which is attached to the femur is chrome cobalt and the materials come from America. It is polished to a high gloss and sterilized before being packed in boxes. They come in 14 different sizes, some wide and some narrow and ones that are not polished are used to insert in the knee to see if it fits before the polished one is inserted. The right and left ones are made differently.

Dr Roger explained that a 'revision' is where the operation is done again. Sometimes the result is not as good as there may be more scar tissue. A 'staged' operation is one that is done after the first one, six months and more apart. 'Bilateral' is where both knees are done simultaneously. We discussed why some people had trouble bending their knees and he said that the scar tissue and the bleeding sometimes prohibited the knee from bending in the early stages.

Dr Roger then took us down to the factory. It was fascinating to see how the different components are made. Huge machines encased in separate compartments do all the work and it takes about two hours for each part and they make about ten in a day. Meticulous care is taken to ensure each component is perfectly sterile. Hydroxy apatite (calcium phosphate or artificial bone) is adhered to the inside of the prosthesis, so that when it is inserted it will be accepted by the knee more readily. I found that fascinating.

The part that will wear out first is the white plastic and that could be replaced at a later date. Much later I hope.

The doctors are not sure how long they will last as this procedure hasn't been around for all that long. They guarantee ten years but maybe 15 or if we're lucky 20 years. Margaret told Dr Roger how much tennis she is playing (around three to four days a week) and he said that the continual rubbing could cause the plastic section to wear down. We asked how we would know if things are wearing out and he replied that the pain would return. Margaret's philosophy is that she wants to enjoy her life now and let the future take care of itself. We could be knocked over by a bus before the knee wears out so get on and do whatever you enjoy doing NOW.

Margaret and I really enjoyed our visit and we now have a better understanding of what goes into a knee replacement. Thank you Dr Greg Roger for showing us around and giving of your time so generously. Let's hope more and more doctors in Australia use your components. After all they are Aussie made and we should support Australian companies if the product is as good as the overseas one. If Dr Merv Cross, the world renowned orthopaedic surgeon uses it surely that is a good enough recommendation.

Dr Merv Cross along with other esteemed doctors did research on comparing Bilateral uncemented Total Knee Arthroplasty and whether simultaneous or staged is better. The report states that 'Patient satisfaction following the bilateral procedure was high. Our average post-op range in the whole cohort is 115 degrees at five years. There are potential and logistic benefits in having simultaneous rather than a staged procedure. Only one anaesthetic is required and hence a reduced operation time. Length of hospital stay has been consistently shown to be the same for uni and bilateral procedures. Physiotherapy and discharge coordination are required only once. It has been shown in the Australian health care system that the out of pocket expenses for the patient are lower than compared with a staged procedure. The exact savings in time and money remain debated.'

They found that 'bilateral procedures have significantly higher rates of complications than unilateral, mainly due to thrombo-embolic problems. This does not however correspond to an increase in mortality rate. If a bilateral procedure is indicated then a simultaneous procedure has no increased risk over a staged one. There is no increase in cardiovascular complications, DVT rate or mortality. The infection rate is lower with a bilateral procedure and the overall revision rate is one percent in all groups. The prosthesis functions as well in bilateral and unilateral procedures in the medium and long term periods.'

To sum it up Dr Cross and his associates came to the conclusion 'that they have no hesitation in supporting the practice of simultaneous bilateral Total Knee Arthroplasty using an uncemented design and feel it is a safe, successful and cost effective strategy for the treatment of bilateral knee arthritis.'

If I had read this report before making up my mind whether to have one done at a time or both together I would have found comfort in these findings. I had age on my side having just turned 64 at the time of my operation. Thank you Dr Cross for allowing me to have access to this report and use some of it in my book.

These facts I found on Dr Cross's web site. 'Of course with any major surgery there can be complications and these include infections, blood clots and the biggest one of all stiffness and not allowing the knee to bend if there is too much swelling around the joint. (As we've heard in some of the letters some patients have to go under anesthetic to get the knee to bend.) Doctors don't like to do knee replacements on patients under 55-60 years due to higher wear and possible need for multiple revisions in their lifetime. Another reason the knee may not bend is bleeding within the joint. Drains are put in to remove the blood but it can sometimes cause problems and delay recovery. It generally responds to ice and physiotherapy.

There also can be nerve injury and this can cause numbness and these areas can be painful and sensitive. It will improve with time.' There is an area on both my knees that is still numb and likely to remain that way for some time.

During this month I decided to put another piece in the *"Insearch"* column of the Daily Telegraph this time asking for people who have had their new knees longer than ten years to e-mail me and tell me how they are now. I also wanted to hear from people who had their knee done again and how they were the second time. Here are some of their letters.

*Dear Pam,*

*In answer to your request in 'In Search', Daily Telegraph, Mon. June 13, my Mum suffered badly from osteo-arthritis and in Dec. 1989, by which time she needed a wheelchair to get around outside the house, she went to have her first knee replacement. She was to have a total replacement of her right knee, however after she had been to theatre her doctor told us he had only done a partial replacement and they had used a new experimental 'glue' for securing the prosthesis. Apart from the wound breaking down, Mum had no real problems with the operation and she was certainly pain free. In Dec. 1990, she went in to have a replacement of her left knee. This also went well and for the first time in years, Mum was completely pain free and able to get around, without having to use a wheelchair. She got ten years good use from her 'new knees', but by 2000, she was beginning to have pains in her knees again and walking was becoming restricted.*

*By 2003, Mum was back to being in a wheelchair and the pain in her knees was a lot worse than she had originally experienced. She saw a new Orthopedic Surgeon who told her, her knee replacements both needed replacing and booked her into hospital. Due to some technical hiccup, Mum's admission was not processed and she was not admitted to hospital. After a lot of hassles, she was finally booked to go in on 5 Oct 2004, to have her right prosthesis replaced, which by this time was causing her continuous pain. However, before this could happen, Mum experienced a near tragedy. On 26 Aug 2004, Mum was admitted to hospital with severe pain in her right knee and was to go to theatre for exploratory surgery. Within a few hours of going to theatre we were called into the hospital as Mum was in Intensive Care in a coma and on haemodialysis as her kidneys had ceased to function and she was not expected to survive. It was a nightmare!*

*The cause of the problem - the partial prosthesis! It had begun to deteriorate and was breaking up and had caused a severe infection which in turn had set up septicaemia throughout her body. It was touch and go but thank goodness with the hard work of the excellent doctors in the Intensive Care Unit, my Mum survived and finally on 3 Feb 2005, after rehabilitation, she went to theatre to have the replacement done. Unfortunately, the wound broke down, but the actual prosthesis the doctors were very happy with. Mum is to go in to have the other knee prosthesis replaced in about three months, but already she is able to get around on a walking frame and at home only uses a walking stick and at 85 years old, we have just taken her and my Dad on a trip to Cairns for a family wedding, which a few months ago we wouldn't have thought would ever be possible! I hope this will be of interest to you and wish you well with both your 'new knees' and your 'new book'!*

*Regards*

*Marie Young*

*PS My Mum's name is Teresa Cook and she lives in Koo We Rup, Victoria and she would be very pleased to have you include her in your book. I live in Macquarie Fields, NSW, a long way to go when your Mum is ill! We, as a family, are very proud of Mum's achievements since she was so critically ill last year, particularly as the doctors were not at all optimistic initially, for even her survival let alone to make the recovery she has. But as Mum says the knee may be good now, but it's all the other body parts that are wearing out after 85 years that are the problem.*

Marie sent the PS when I replied to her and asked permission to include her Mum's story. What a brave lady! I can't believe that a half knee caused all those problems. Doing my maths the knees were replaced 16 years ago but she began having trouble at the ten year mark. So what Dr Roger told us is true, that pain will tell us when it's time to have them done again. It's a shame she had to wait a further five years before getting relief in one knee at least. She is about to have her second one replaced. We wish her well and hopefully with no complications.

*Hi Pam,*
*My father, Spencer Greer, is 89. He had his 1st knee replacement is 1989, his 2nd in 1990. Everything was fine. In 1999 he had further surgery to replace a part that had worn out in his right knee. The surgery was successful, but two days after returning home the local doctor found that my father was suffering from an infection. It took several days in hospital to discover what this infection actually was. He subsequently spent eight weeks in hospital with total bed rest. It was then found that the cruciate ligament was no longer viable. He is now taking antibiotics for the rest of his life to counteract the infection. The only alternative is to take out the prosthesis and leave him with a stiff leg. He now wears a leg brace permanently. He was never a particularly active man due to a bad back but now finds that he cannot even shower himself without help. Home Care come in every day to help with his shower but unfortunately Veterans Affairs refuse to help with any improvements to the bathroom to help.*
*Hope this information assists.*
*Regards,*
*Lesley Haynes (daughter)*

Lesley's father also had ten years out of his knee replacement. It is 16 years since he first had it done and in that time improvements have been made in the procedure. Infections are a worry and it was dreadful that it happened in Spencer's case. I'm sorry to hear he now has to wear a brace and has to have help. At least he had ten years of being pain free. Otherwise, he may have been in a wheelchair had he not been able to have a knee replacement. We have to be thankful we live in these times where this type of surgery is available. Of course we're all living longer so it is inevitable that certain parts of our bodies will wear out.

*Dear Pam,*
*I was booked in to have a right knee replacement at Manly Hospital on 11 February 2001. My ordeal began before the operation as I was prepared for theatre in the morning but not taken until four in the afternoon, all that time without sedation, food or drink.*

*The operation went without a hitch and I was still under the effects of the anesthetic all night but by morning the pain was excruciating. I was told to press a button for morphine to be released into a saline drip but no matter how often I pressed it didn't seem to make any difference to the pain. I was left in bed all day but the next day the physiotherapist appeared and I had to get out of bed to exercise the knee. Another totally unexpected amount of pain! In fact I screamed so loudly that I was left in peace. It was the same for the following days and I was warned that I would end up with a stiff leg. By that time I was beyond caring about anything but the pain.*

*I was discharged after one week with tramal capsules for the pain which worked a lot better than the morphine drip. At home I could take as many Panadols as I liked. The pain went on for six weeks. I had a low temperature on and off and found it very hard to do the exercises and could not attend the physio department at Manly Hospital for five weeks.*

*Just as I thought I was over the worst I was summoned back to see my doctor urgently. I was totally unprepared for what was to follow. My doctor told me that the operation would have to be repeated as the lower part had refused to heal onto the bone due to a faulty transplant manufactured by a company in a European country. A whole batch was bad and some 50 people in Australia suffered the same fate. A white line on the X-ray showed the gap between the implant and the bone and without another operation the knee would be unsteady forever.*

*So I had another operation at the Mater Hospital on 1 July 2001. The pain was controlled by Panadeine Forte by mouth which was a lot better than the drip the first time. This enabled me to do the exercises although it took several weeks before I could move the knee properly. My doctor was very helpful and came to see me the night before the second operation to make sure I could face another one. This time it was all so much better, probably because only half needed to be done and because the implant was not faulty. My body must have rejected the faulty one because it caused so much pain, much more than other people seem to have suffered.*

*All is well after four years. The knee is movable back and forward without pain but a pin had to be put in the bottom section to strengthen the bone that had broken when the prosthesis was removed. I do hope that doesn't cause me too much bother in years to come.*

Name withheld because this lady received compensation from the company and doesn't want the world to know. This same company had to pay compensation to over 3000 hip and knee replacements in America. A bit scary!

*Dear Pam,*

*Two years ago I had a knee replacement done which caused me considerable pain for 12 months afterwards. I paid monthly visits to my surgeon and had numerous X-rays done but at the end of 12 months, the pain did not subside. It was at this point that the surgeon told me about the company who made the prosthesis were having similar trouble with their implants with other people as well.*

*A year ago I booked into a private hospital at the expense of this company and had the procedure done again. It was thought that the first time failed because of the wrong compound used in the operation. All my expenses were paid for including physiotherapy afterwards but I didn't get the same movement back which I had before the operation. It seems that each time you have a replacement you lose more bend in your knee.*

*As it stands now I am still waiting for a claim on pain and suffering which the company has promised to pay.*

*Henny Cahill*

Henny is a member of my writing group and offered to tell her story. She has suffered a great deal and now faces another operation on her other knee. She is not looking forward to having to go through it all again. Good luck Henny, may you sail through the next one with no complications. At least you know what to expect.

*Hello Pam,*

*I am 5′6″ and weigh 61kg. I have skinny knees, knock knees and pigeon-toed. From an early age I excelled at sport especially running, sprinting and hockey and anything else that was going. I just loved sport generally. Saturdays from an early age was sport, sport, sport. I did a lot of sprinting until the age of 14 and continued hockey (until my knee trouble), cricket and I enjoyed five and ten km fun runs which I now know was very hard on my knees and caused a lot of harm.*

*I remember the day I was full flight down the left-wing playing hockey when my right knee gave way and I didn't play hockey again. I was then 39 years old. For the next four years I had X-rays, arthroscopes and even had acupuncture. I went to Sydney and had radioactive gold injected into my knee to try to curtail the pain. By this time my knee was down to bone on bone. I was trying to keep my part time cleaning job as well as trying to keep sane with the pain.*

*Finally, after convincing my orthopedic surgeon that my whole personality was changing because of the pain, that I was constantly cranky and very hard to get along with, he agreed to do the first replacement of my right knee. I was 43 at the time. This was performed in 1993 at Tamara Private Hospital in Tamworth. The actual operation was straight forward but I was badly let down by my physio who was an older lady and though she walked me a lot, she did not encourage much bending. I was very naïve. Consequently, I left hospital without even a 90 degree bend. I then went to a private physio for some time but the scar tissue had set in and I never achieved a decent result.*

*By 1999 my left knee was troubling me and the only answer was total knee replacement. This one was successful and with hard work, a lot of determination and a very dedicated physio a much better bend was achieved. I have not been able to run or kneel since my replacements but I love to walk and take my brown miniature poodle Jock daily. I am still a trifle envious when the annual Tamworth Fun Run comes around but these thoughts pass and I am content again.*

*Only about four months ago I started to experience pain at the base of my right knee extending to the calf muscle. The physio suggested that the cement may have loosened and so off I went to see an orthopedic surgeon at the North Sydney Orthopedic and Sports Centre. He ordered blood tests and a nuclear scan. The diagnosis was exactly as the physio had thought and the only answer was a revision knee replacement. This will be a much bigger operation as he will have to take out the old prosthesis and scrape out all the old cement but I am confident of a good result.*

*This will take place next Monday 27 June at the Mater Hospital and I am hopeful I will get a good movement this time as I am much more experienced now and know what to expect. I believe the result depends a lot on me and the work I put into my physio. You asked how I knew I needed replacements. With the first one it was dramatic pain, a lot of noise, movement, clicking etc. With the second, not as dramatic but a lot of pain. Now with the revision about to happen at first only slight pain and after a couple of months painful cramping especially at night when my leg was relaxed.*

*Hope this info can help.*

*Regards,*

*Di Hodgins*

Di, your letter contains a lot of helpful advice. You had 12 years out of your first replacement before having to have it done again. Let's hope the second one lasts even longer. Your story is one that will be repeated over and over with the number of young ones playing so much sport. Orthopedic surgeons will be kept busy for years to come. My brother David was also a keen sportsman; cricket and football being his sports. Of course over time the knees began to wear out as did his shoulders. He has had one operation on his shoulder and now a new procedure on his knee. (Since writing he has had a second new shoulder performed. He is truly the bionic man.) Below is his story.

*In previous times, when the knee cap was stuck hard to the knee with no movement, they simply removed the kneecap! I had a new procedure called Patella Semoral Arthroplasty whereby a small rubber prosthesis is inserted under the kneecap to give movement to the old knee. It involved a cut of some six inches at the edge of the kneecap, lifting it up and inserting the prosthesis. I was on crutches for only three days. Full recovery is six to eight weeks for full movement. At my stage, four weeks on Thursday, it is still sore but after much icing, heat and exercise I can walk up and down stairs and walk OK. As it softens up I should come good completely. It was an expensive operation for me as my health fund did not cover knees and I'm $7000 out of pocket!*
*David Jolly*

The procedure is certainly a much quicker one as David was only in hospital one day. I'll be very interested in his full recovery. I don't think David had top cover with his health fund so if you want this done it is worth checking with your fund first. His procedure cost him the same as my two knees and I was in hospital for much longer. He assures me it will last a long time and he won't need a knee replacement in the future. I hope this is true.

*Dear Pam,*
*I am 80 years old, well almost 80. I had my first knee replacement in 1990 and second in 1992. Both operations were not quite what you would call successful. I had opinions by Swiss, Czech and Australian orthopedic surgeons. Their verdict was: in perfect order. I had a follow check up by the Melbourne surgeon some two years ago as he and other surgeons tried to find out the problem that I and some 1% or 2% of patients who have similar post operatic problems, have experienced. Unfortunately there is no improvement. I suffer from acute stiffness. These days I walk, not very far with a walking stick.*
*George Korda*

George has certainly had his knees a long time but I'm sorry to hear they have been not too good. As he said some have to be in the bottom two percent. Sorry it had to be George.

*Dear Pam,*

*My first knee replacement, the right one, (the worst one first) was done at Bathurst Hospital by a young, enthusiastic, energetic Orthopedic Specialist, Dr David Daniel O'Keefe who had come there as a locum for the resident surgeon to have leave. My left knee followed eight months later, July 1986, same hospital, same surgeon. I think he told me it was the first uncemented one done in that hospital. A most wonderful exercise machine was used in bed on the third day. It automatically bent the knee for the required time. It was in great demand and had to be shared.*

*Lots of physio at our local hospital followed and though there is still some stiffness, there is NO pain and I have never had a problem. I wish you every success with your book and your own replacement.*

*Yours sincerely,*

*Rita Slattery.*

I spoke to Rita on the phone before getting her letter and I enjoyed speaking to her. She is now in her eighties and had her knees done when she was in her sixties. The fact that hers were uncemented all those years ago is interesting. They have lasted 20 years and are still going strong. She told me she wouldn't allow me to use the name of her doctor without getting his permission first. She did some detective work to find where this doctor is now practising. After many phone calls she finally tracked him down and he was living not too far away in Orange on a property. Rita lives in Cowra. Dr O'Keefe is no longer practising medicine after two unfortunate accidents. He was most interested to hear that Rita's knees were still going well after all this time. He was only in his early thirties when he did the operation all those years ago. He asked her if she had had any X-rays taken in that time and Rita said no. So he's going to arrange with her doctor to have it done to see how they are now.

Rita was very excited when she phoned to tell me she had found her doctor and he had given permission to use his name in my story. I still wanted to know where he had learnt to use the uncemented version of the knee replacement. Rita gave me his number so I rang him myself. He told me he trained at the Newcastle District Hospital. At the time Rita was told by others that it was a risk doing it this way as most were cemented in the early days. Who has had the last laugh? I asked Rita in one of our phone calls how energetic she had been during the 20 years and she had to admit she wasn't overly active. In other words she didn't play a sport and so hasn't done anything dramatic to wear them out. Perhaps the ones playing sport may not get the 20 years but here's hoping.

I was also interested in the machine that was used at Bathurst Hospital to bend the knee and so rang my doctor to see why I didn't see one at the Mater or Delmar hospitals. His secretary told me that some doctors use them but mine didn't believe it helped very much. So the jury is out on that one. Rita has now had her X-ray and the results were sent to Dr O'Keefe who consulted with other orthopedic surgeons in the area and found that Rita's knees are in fine shape. They will surely outlive her. Here is Dr O'Keefe's reply to me.

*Dear Pam,*
*Having been retired from active orthopedic practice for over five years now, a call from an old patient can send cold shivers down your spine with thoughts of 'What's gone wrong?' and 'who's going to fix it now that you can't' etc. I was pleasantly surprised to hear from Rita who is now 85 years old and living in a nearby rural town in NSW. She told me that I had performed two knee replacements on her at Bathurst Hospital in 1985 when I was a 'keen young surgeon'; and that they are both still going very nicely after 20 years!*

*When I picked myself up off the floor I asked her a few more questions and it would seem that although she never achieved more than 90 degrees bend in either of them, she could still walk to the shop and do her own domestic chores, although she admits to not being as sprightly as she once was. Suspecting that this might be a similar circumstance to the second-hand car dealer who will tell you that 'it was only owned by a little old lady who drove it to church on Sundays', despite the fact that it's very ancient. I asked Rita if she would have some Xrays and send them to me as I wasn't even certain what prosthesis I had used back in 1985.*

*After a few weeks the films arrived and to my astonishment they were two of the original PCA uncemented knees (you remember - the ones with the single screw and two oblique studs for tibial fixation and a metal backed patella). I discussed the films with my colleagues at the recent meeting of the Western Orthopedic Group in Orange; and the general consensus was that they would normally expect about a ten year longevity for this prosthesis. All the major components retain their position with some narrowing of the poly on the medial side of both knees, with some minor subsidence of the tibial component on the left. There looks to be excellent bony ingrowth / ongrowth to the two tibial lugs on both (they were porous coated). The lateral views are not as com-plimentary however, showing evidence of superior migration of both the patellar components and some anterior tilting of the left tibial tray with marked sclerosis, but the component still appears to be stable. I note that as the operations were carried out some months apart that the type of screws used were different and the femoral component on the left is at least one size smaller than the one used on the right.*

*Still and all, 'the proof of the pudding is in the eating' and they have lasted her 20 years and she remains very happy with them. I asked her how much longer she planned to keep using them and the answer was much less specific, but we both agreed that they would 'last her out'!*

*In the light of what we now know about tibial fixation and polyethylene thickness, not to mention the infamous metal-backed patella, one could hardly imagine that two of these early uncemented knee prostheses would last as long as they have. Rita attributes their success to the skill of the young and keen surgeon and whilst not wanting to disillusion her too much on that point, I would have to say that the word 'SERENDIPITY' comes immediately to mind!*

*Regards,*
*Dr Danny O'Keefe*

Dr O'Keefe kindly sent me Rita's X-rays and this is how they were done 20 years ago. The obvious difference is that they were uncemented and the other orthopedic surgeons who looked at these X-rays were amazed they had lasted so long. Lucky for you Rita that Dr O'Keefe came into your life all those years ago.

I would like to thank all those people who replied to my second "*Insearch*" request. The information received I hope will give more insight into the long-term outcome.

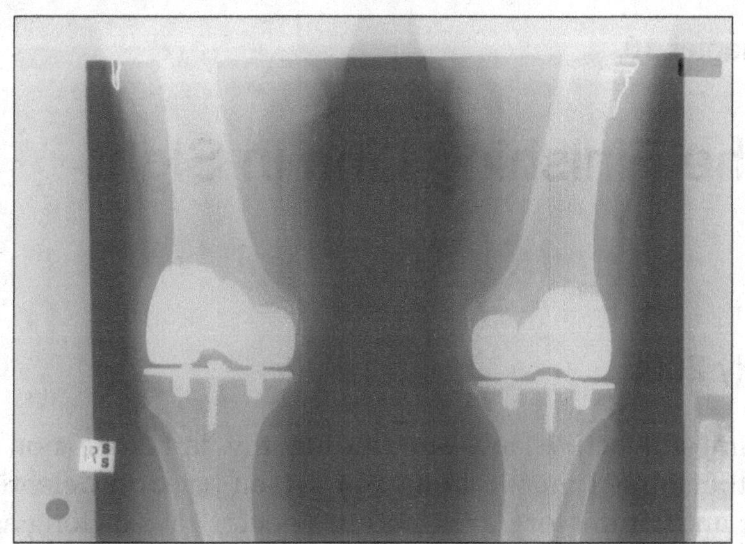

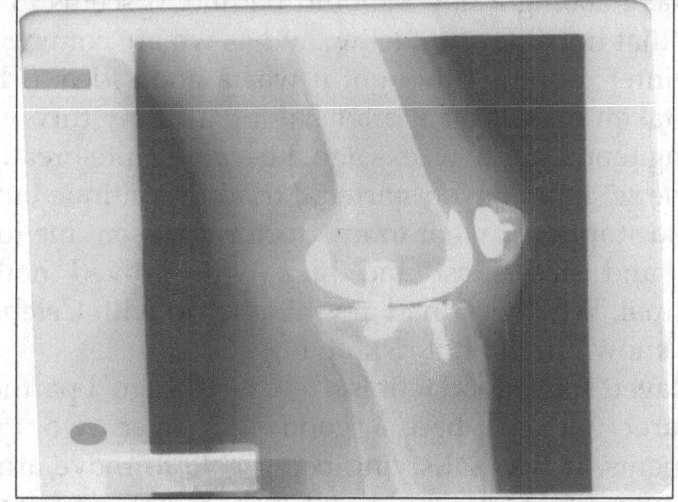

**Rita's X-rays.**

Chapter 10

# The Finishing Line in Sight

## July 2005

I am still active and am finding my left knee not so bothersome. I must admit I put myself back on Celebrex, the antiflammatory drug and my doctor says as long as I only take 200mg a day I should be fine. It seems to take away that horrible stiff feeling and as we are coming into the winter months I thought it was a good idea. (I have since taken myself off it after having a funny turn while playing tennis a few weeks ago. I became quite breathless and the set hadn't even started. I tried to continue but felt faint so stopped. I went to my doctor who sent me for an X-ray and stress test and they both proved nothing abnormal. Whether it had anything to do with Celebrex I don't know but I'm not risking it.)

I played some good tennis a few weeks ago. I partnered Margaret and we had a good win over two tough opponents. It was satisfying being able to move around the court. Before I would call out 'Yours' and let my partner do all the running. Now they are making up for all that slack time and are making me work hard. Keep it up girls, I need to feel wanted.

The 'New Knees Club' is alive and thriving. Norma came up for a game recently and she is back to her old form. Of course she had only a half knee replacement. We keep rubbing that in. Bev is going really well and is playing the best tennis I've seen her play in a long time. Her backhand passing shots are killers.

Jan is now a grandmother to a baby girl and she's delighted. Her daughter Nicole gave birth three weeks ago and Ashley is a lucky girl to have her grandmother living next door. They will form a beautiful bond. Jan will be too busy minding the baby to be able to join us on the tennis court. The other girls in my tennis group, Faye, Peg, Helena, and Carolyn have not had any knee problems and I certainly hope they don't get any. Nola hasn't been able to play with us for a while and is deciding what to do about her knees. The doctor says they are not bad enough for knee replacements yet. We miss you Nola.

I thank my new knees every day as I've had a lot of walking to do to visit my mother in hospital during three different stays recently. Remarkably she pulled through each one and is back in her own little unit in her assisted living retirement village. She is after all nearly 93. Garnet's mother died in March aged 98, six weeks short of her 99th birthday. We all thought she would make 100 but a broken hip put paid to that goal.

I have an exciting year ahead as my son Justin is getting married to Karla in October at Lake Tahoe in California. Garnet, Mark and I are going over but Cameron and Nadia will have a brand new baby by then (now born and it is a beautiful little girl called Sofia) and will be a little busy. Thank goodness I had my operation when I did as I'll be able to enjoy all the activities that are on offer. I will also be seeing my best friend Chris Machado who lives in San Diego on the way home. I haven't seen Chris in quite a while so it will be fun catching up. We used to play tennis together at Manly Lawn when our boys were small. She has a Justin as well.

Tomorrow I go for my 12 monthly check up. I'm having some X-rays done and then I go to see Dr Walter. I hope he's going to say my knees are fine and just get on with your life. I can hardly believe that a year has slipped by and so much has happened. I am glad I had both done together even though the rehab took a bit longer but in the long run it's pleasing to know I don't have to go back and go through it all again for a few years at least. Hopefully 15-20 will be good and by then medical science will have improved on the procedure. I'm not in any pain. I can walk up and down stairs without any difficulty, play tennis to a reasonable standard and go for long walks which I love.

I arrive early for my X-rays which are over in a flash. I wait to take them with me. Dr Walter's surgery is on the same level. I still have half an hour before my appointment time so I read my book. I walk in ten minutes before my appointed time and am asked to fill in a form. I recognise it as the one I filled in the first time I came to see Dr Walter. It asks questions about your pain level four weeks prior, doing all sorts of things e.g. walking upstairs, shopping, sleeping etc. and I can fill in the no pain square for everyone without hesitation. I turn the page over and there it asks post operation questions and I can confidently say how good my knees are. I do mention that my left one is a bit tight and that both are stiff from time to time. I give an eight out of ten satisfaction rating.

I'm called in and up on the screen are my X-rays. I look at them closely. I can't believe those big chunks are in my knees. His assistant chats to me and then Dr Walter walks in. He looks at the X-rays and smiles.

'They look pretty good to me. How have they been?'

'I'm back playing tennis, doctor and I'm actually running for lobs.' I then proceed to tell him about the book I'm writing and ask permission to use his name which he gives. He also asks if he can read the manuscript before publishing it and I agree. He asks me to show him how I'm walking and then he examines me. He bends my knees and says they are both bending about the same. He's pleased with how strong they are and tells me they should last 15-20 years. Let's hope he's right! That will make me about 85. That seems a long way off.

Dr Walter then asks me if I am glad I had them both done together and I say yes. There were times when I may have given a different answer but it is so comforting to know I don't have to return to have the other one done. I did say that it was the uncertainty of what I was facing that made it so terrifying. Maybe it's not so daunting the second time around.

I walk out of his surgery with a big smile on my face. I can remember thinking I'd never reach this milestone when I was in agony and finding it so hard to bend my knees in the first weeks. Life is kind and time does move on and the memories are fading (except when I read my book over and over in the editing stage).

So my advice is, if you are in constant pain and life is unbearable go and have your knees replaced. You will never be sorry as many of the letters testify. Let's all hope we can be like Rita who has had hers for 20 years and has had no trouble with them. She is an inspiration. I want to be like her.

# EPILOGUE

I have just returned from two weeks in America. I was there for my son's wedding to his beautiful bride Karla. Having two good knees certainly made a big difference to the enjoyment of this holiday. It is amazing how much walking you have to do. Boarding planes, moving from one terminal to another, sightseeing, looking at shops, climbing up small ladders as we had to do when visiting the aircraft carrier Midway and all the hundreds of other things you do when you're on vacation.

The first four days were spent in San Francisco where we saw the naval air show and that involved a lot of walking around Fisherman's Wharf. My knees got a good work out that day. The bus tour around the city was a highlight of our trip and the weather was perfect. In fact most of the time the weather was kind to us. Riding on the cable car was an experience and some mad fools love hanging off it as it climbs the steep streets of the city.

We hired a car to take us to Lake Tahoe and driving across the Oakland Bay bridge in peak hour, on the opposite side of the road, was a frightening experience. Maybe more so for my dear husband who told me later how terrified he was! We met up with the bride and groom in Reno and picked up youngest son Mark at the airport. Justin and Karla were staying at a casino for three nights and would drive to Tahoe the next day. Mark travelled with us and was staying at the same place as us.

The wedding was three days away and so we had time to look around and get our bearings. Justin and Karla had planned an outdoor wedding with the tall peaked mountains and the lake in the background. As it was autumn the leaves were changing colour and looked magnificent. I have never seen such a glorious setting for a wedding. The size of the lake and the reflection of the mountains shimmering on the glassy surface were breathtaking.

The day before the wedding the forecast was for a cold snap with the possibility of snow. Karla had to hastily change the arrangements. A chapel in one of the casinos where her parents were staying was chosen and the only time we could have was 11.30am, which meant a four hour wait for the reception.

The day of the wedding dawned. As I looked out the door, to my great surprise snowflakes began to flutter down, later followed by a heavy dump of snow. It looked so pretty but our main concern was how we were going to get our car out of the steep driveway. A large four wheeled drive came down, leaving huge tracks in the snow which Garnet followed. After getting my hair done we were on our way after picking up Justin at his hotel. Karla had left much earlier to meet up with her mother and bridesmaids for the usual pampering.

I have never seen a more beautiful bride and I was a proud mother that day seeing my eldest son marry his sweetheart with whom he had been living the last four years. Justin looked handsome in his dinner suit, blue vest and tie. Cameras clicked merrily the whole day. After the ceremony the couple went outside for more photos and it was very cold. Karla had a fur lined jacket to put around her shoulders and she needed it. She looked so pretty.

The reception was at a restaurant which had magnificent views of the lake, a great setting for more photos. This was only a small wedding - just Karla's family, ours and a few friends. An enjoyable time was had by all. Garnet and I had the honour of travelling back to our hotel in the married couple's eight seated limousine.

We ended our American holiday with four days in San Diego staying with friends. I'm so glad I went and I kept thinking to myself how lucky I was that I had had my knee operation the year before. I could never have managed to do all the things I did with my old knees. I would have been a drag on everyone. On the plane I made sure I got up every so often and wriggled my toes a lot. On the return flight I requested a seat with more leg room as on the inward flight I had found it very difficult to move my legs at all.

I hope you have learnt something from my experiences and if I have helped one person overcome the fear of having a knee replacement this book has been worthwhile. Just remember it is painful and you think you will never be any good again, but you will.

www.ingramcontent.com/pod-product-compliance
Lightning Source LLC
LaVergne TN
LVHW030912080826
845145LV00010B/2862